Under the Drapes:

More Mystique of Surgery

by David Gelber, MD

RUFFIANPRESS

Ruffian Press
150 FM 1959
Houston, TX 77034
www.ruffianpress.com
www.itpfuturehope.com

Library of Congress Control Number: 2012909703

ISBN-13 978-0-9820763-6-1
ISBN-10 09820763-6-3

First Edition - 2012

Cover Image: http://www.123rf.com/photo_6137312
Cover Design: Elizabeth E. Little, Hyliian Designs
http://hyliian.deviantart.com

Typesetting/Book Layout Design:
Ellen C. Maze, The Author's Mentor
www.theauthorsmentor.com

Printed in the United States of America

Dedication

This book is dedicated to Laura, my beautiful, loving, understanding wife of 26 years who has endured innumerable solitary nights and untimely interruptions with patience and a smile.

Under the Drapes:

More Mystique of Surgery

by David Gelber, MD

Contents

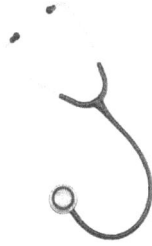

1. Why do you do it?

Do what? Get up in the middle of the night? Rush in to the hospital to patch mangled bodies, sew holes closed, stick my finger in a dike spewing blood and, hopefully, repair what's broken and allow some unfortunate soul to live and love another day? A good question. I could have been a pediatrician, almost became one as a matter of fact, or a plastic surgeon, but I failed the ego test. No, I had to be a general surgeon... for glory? No. For personal satisfaction? Maybe. For intellectual stimulation? Perhaps. For the money? Definitely not. Then...why?

Why did I go to school for all those years? Elementary school, junior high school, senior high school, four years of college, four years of medical school, five years of residency, working a hundred hours a week? All for what? To be able to wrestle with an intoxicated man at 3:00 a.m., trying to evaluate the stab wound to his buttock or fathom why a beautiful woman would decide, in a moment of severe, devastating depression, that she didn't like her breasts and tried to cut them off? Or why a distraught father failed to check behind his car as he pulled out of his driveway, just to pick up a container of milk, and inadvertently ran over his 2-year-old daughter?

Why do bowels perforate, aneurysms burst, appendices rupture, arteries clog, gallstones form; why does anything bad have to happen? Why do the nicest people you could ever meet develop inoperable and incurable stomach cancer; why does anyone have to get cancer? Can't we do something to prevent it?

You ask why I do it. Can anyone answer even one of these questions or a million other, similar ones?

But, every illness, all the injuries, all the misguided thoughts and actions, every trivial, little act that we wish we could take back, every moment that should never have happened, all these things that bring us to a doctor seeking a remedy, are they reasons enough? The battle against disease rages onward, fought by doctors, nurses, technicians, and therapists at all hours of the day and night; most of the time the battle is won, but the war always goes on, never ending. And if it never ends, if there can be no victory, what's the point?

Is it enough to replace the look of overwhelming fear and distress, a look I routinely see on patients' (and their families') faces, with a smile? Is the look of relief on the faces of worried family members when they are told that everything went well, that the lump was benign, that the injuries are not severe, that their son will be back on the basketball court in just a few weeks, enough reward?

I've asked myself these questions over and over again. Sometimes I have the answer; sometimes I just shake my head in bewilderment; but all the time I answer the call, do my best, and hope that those I try to help, the sick and injured, return to a normal life.

So I come to the hospital at 3:00 a.m. and probe and palpate and listen and probe some more. And then, I cut and dissect and clamp and tie and cauterize and sew and resect and reanastamose and bypass and sew some more. All of this so that, in the end, a person, broken by the struggles of life in this fallen world, can have a few more moments as a complete individual.

Why do I do it? Because of what's waiting for me under those drapes. A patient, with a name and a family, who has entrusted me with their very being. But...do I deserve such trust?

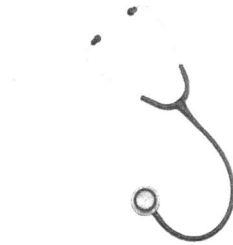

2. Why Do Surgery?

"I feel the capacity to care is the thing which gives life its deepest significance."

~ Pablo Casals

1. Treat Infection - Drain Abscesses, Control Fistulas, Remove Necrotic Tissue

2. Relieve Obstruction - Blockage of Intestine, Bile Ducts, Pancreas, etc.

3. Restore Circulation - Remove or Bypass Thromboses or Atherosclerosis; Repair Traumatic Occlusions

4. Remove Tumors - Benign or Malignant

5. Repair Injuries - Trauma to any body part, orthopedic, ophthalmic, neurologic, etc.

6. Reconstruction of Injured, Damaged or Excised Tissue or Organs - Post Cancer surgery, Post

radiation therapy, Post severe infection or trauma.

7. Restore Cosmesis - Congenital or Acquired Deformity

8. Control Bleeding - Post Trauma, Post Intervention or Spontaneous

9. Diagnose Pathologic Processes - Biopsy of Tumors, Excision of Lymph Nodes

10. Allow Access for Therapeutic Intervention - Venous, Arterial, Peritoneal, Thoracic, or Intrathecal Access

11. 11. Replace Severely Damaged Organs - Transplant Surgery, Total Joint Replacement

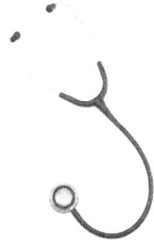

3. Flowing

Our bodies are molded rivers.

~ Novalis

The human body is an amazing biological machine, composed of a series of parallel conduits which carry materials to and from its various end organs. Proper functioning of this incredible apparatus depends on uninterrupted flow through these pipes. Disruption of this normal flow usually leads to dysfunction of the end organ, followed by the development of symptoms, ultimately sending the suffering individual to the doctor's office or Emergency Room (ER) at the local hospital.

Almost every cell depends on unimpeded flow to deliver important supplies, whether from an internal gland or organ, or from the world outside. From the top of the body, in our head, to our backside and through to our toes, materials flow through an enormous network of tubes and ducts, bringing essential resources in and carrying waste products out. Organ systems are interconnected by this vast array of conduits: the heart, a tireless pump, sends blood under high pressure through arteries to every muscle, organ, nerve, and bone, while veins carry the depleted, deoxygenated blood back to the heart; capillaries are very fine vessels that connect the arteries to the veins, dropping off essential nutrients and picking up the cellular garbage, to be carried to the kidney, lungs and skin to be eliminated; nerves are bioelectrical sensors and activators that modulate a wide variety of actions; a variety of duct work connects one organ to another; lymphatics carry fluids that the blood vessels can't; exocrine glands send their products through ducts to be delivered to a specific area; endocrine glands dump their products directly into the bloodstream to be delivered to the entire body; intestines keep ingested materials moving through us, absorbing what's necessary, while ignoring the rest; airways bring the good air in and eliminate the bad air and its metabolic byproducts. Most of these pipes have some sort of control mechanism or are adaptable to a variability in the flow of materials. Veins come with valves to keep blood flowing toward the heart; sphincters exist at various points along our gastrointestinal (GI) tract to help modulate flow of ingested food and digestive enzymes, allowing for orderly processing of nutrients; many of these passageways can dilate or constrict, depending on the dynamics of flow. But, no matter which conduit one considers, the malfunction, obstruction, or disruption of flow can cause serious, sometimes life-threatening illness.

Starting at the top, the lacrimal gland secretes tears which bathe our eyes and are then collected in the lacrimal duct where the tears flow into our pharynx. Salivary glands produce saliva, which passes through a duct and into our mouth, aiding digestion by moistening and softening the food we consume. Saliva also maintains lubrication of our mouth and pharynx, keeping us comfortable, and preventing our tongue from sticking to the roof of our mouth. Obstruction of lacrimal ducts or salivary glands leads to symptoms that often require surgical intervention, by an ophthalmologist or otolaryngologist.

The salivary glands and lacrimal glands are examples of exocrine glands. They secrete materials that pass through ducts, into a recipient end organ, in these examples, eyes, and pharynx. Other exocrine glands are the digestive portion of the pancreas, biliary system of the liver, and sweat glands of the skin. Interruption to free flow in any one of these glands can cause symptoms and, particularly in the liver or pancreas, sometimes life-threatening inflammation or infection.

The obstruction of ducts originating in the liver or pancreas and draining into the duodenum almost always leads to hospitalization and a visit from a general surgeon. Pancreatic obstruction causes pancreatitis which can be a simple, transient phenomenon caused by the passage of a gallstone, or it can be a life-threatening condition that requires a prolonged stay in an Intensive Care Unit (ICU). The blockage of the pancreas causes the digestive enzymes to "back up" in the pancreas and leak out into the surrounding tissues, and these enzymes begin to digest the normal tissue. In severe cases, the nearby intestine might be affected, leading to a fistula; or blood vessels might be weakened, causing bleeding, so-called "Hemorrhagic Pancreatitis," the most serious type of pancreatic inflammation, which is often fatal.

Biliary tract obstruction can be just as serious. If the gallbladder becomes obstructed, most commonly by gallstones, treatment is usually straightforward: remove the gallbladder along with the offending stone(s). If the main bile ducts, those that allow bile to drain from the liver and/or gallbladder into the duodenum (first part of the small intestine), become blocked, the individual usually becomes jaundiced, manifested by yellowish discoloration of the skin, most noticeable in the whites of the eyes. Infection of the obstructed bile duct by bacteria results in life-threatening sepsis, secondary to a condition called "ascending cholangitis." Untreated, this condition has nearly 100% mortality. Rapid intervention with appropriate antibiotics and relief of the obstruction is necessary. Unblocking the bile duct always requires some procedural intervention, be it surgical, endoscopic, or radiologic.

General Surgeons are frequently called out to attend to patients with intestinal obstruction, sometimes mechanical and sometimes functional. No matter what the cause, the interruption to normal flow causes symptoms, symptoms designed to clearly tell the sick individual that something is definitely amiss. Severe abdominal pains, intense cramping, nausea and vomiting, and severe constipation, (termed obstipation), are the hallmarks of mechanical intestinal obstruction. The cause varies from simple adhesions (scar tissue from previous surgery or inflammation), which can lead to twisting or kinking of this flexible tube of bowels; tumors which can obstruct from within, like waste or debris clogging a sewer line, or from without, akin to the roots of a tree growing into a pipe (time to call Roto-Rooter); foreign objects can become lodged within our bowels; sometimes the bowel becomes narrowed by inflammation or poor blood supply. So many things can cause obstruction, but they all have one thing in common: a complete and persistent obstruction necessitates some sort of intervention, usually surgery, to provide relief and restore the normal flow of intestinal contents.

An adhesion is scar tissue that develops after a previous surgery or secondary to an inflammatory condition, resulting in two structures being bound together. Bowel obstruction due to adhesions is caused by bowels getting wrapped around these adhesions or herniating through areas involved with adhesions, causing kinks, constriction, or twisting. Surgery for adhesions involves cutting away the scar tissue to remove the source of blockage. This might involve snipping a single adhesive band, which might take only a few minutes, or it might require hours of dissection. The point of obstruction is usually clearly identifiable. The obstructed bowel is dilated, blown up like a balloon as air and GI contents back up from the point of obstruction. Beyond this point the bowels are collapsed.

The discrepancy sometimes is very striking. An obstructed bowel might be 5 or 6 or more centimeters (cm) in diameter with a bluish hue caused by congested veins; the unobstructed bowel, which has emptied itself of all its contents, is pink and shriveled up, sometimes looking like a decorative ribbon barely 1 cm in diameter. Once the point of obstruction is identified, the surgeon must decide how to handle the problem. A single adhesive band usually poses no dilemma; snip it away, look at the bowel and be sure that it has adequate circulation and is not compromised in any way. More adhesions might require a more complex procedure. Sometimes the intestines are a solid mass, adhesions causing the bowels to be glued together into a huge blob. Carving the bowel free from dense adhesions often leaves several segments of bowel that appear ragged and torn. Usually repairs can be made; the bowel will heal surprisingly well. However, sometimes the bowel will look so extremely ragged that repairs are not feasible and resection (removal) of a segment becomes necessary. This increases the potential for complications. An obstructed bowel is commonly overgrown with bacteria; any spillage can lead to serious infection. There is also the possibility that the anastamosis (connection) will not heal.

The course of action depends on a large number of variables: What is the patient's overall condition? What is their nutritional state? Is there likely to be ongoing infection or has the source been completely removed? Are there any concerns about blood supply to the affected area? What part of the bowel is involved? A patient with an obstructed, perforated colon with massive intraperitoneal contamination, and multiple abscesses with signs of severe sepsis is at high risk for poor healing and would best be served by removal of the offending bowel and creation of a colostomy. At the other end of the spectrum, a young healthy man who has an ischemic segment of jejunum, caused by adhesions from the stab wound he suffered three years before, can safely have the bad segment resected and reanastamosed with the expectation of complete and uncomplicated recovery.

What about impedance to flow in other systems? Volumes of books have been written about blockages in arteries and veins. Each side of the circulatory system presents a unique set of problems. Arterial obstruction might cause symptoms ranging from none, or transient pain, up to gangrene and necrosis; it all depends on whether the blockage occurs suddenly or over a long period of time and if there is collateral circulation. Arteries are all two-way streets; the direction of blood flow depends on the pressure gradients that exist within the vessel. Typically, blood flows from larger arteries to smaller, more distal ones as the pressure generated in the heart pushes the blood into arteries, then arterioles, then capillaries, and finally into the venous circulation.

If an artery becomes blocked, a thrombus, or clot, will develop within the lumen of the vessel and will extend back to a point where unimpeded flow can occur, often to a bifurcation or site of a large collateral vessel. Thus, the blood can flow around the blocked artery via side streets or collateral vessels. If, however, the artery is what's called an end artery and the only blood supply to an organ, then occlusion of that artery invariably leads to damage. The kidney is an example of an end organ; occlusion of the renal artery leads to infarction of the kidney. The stomach, on the other hand, has arterial supply from four different arteries and a rich supply of collaterals, making infarction resulting from occlusion of one of its supplying arteries unlikely.

Even if arterial flow is not completely disrupted, only diminished, the end organ and its owner still might suffer. Angina, or chest pain, results from heart muscle that is deprived of adequate oxygen due to diminished blood flow, usually caused by narrowing of arteries. Intermittent claudication is pain in the legs that occurs during walking. The increased energy demands associated with activity cannot be met by the diminished arterial flow through a narrowed vessel, and the muscles start to ache. Usually such pain occurs after walking a certain distance and is relieved by rest. The underlying disorder is a tight narrowing or complete blockage of one of the major arteries in the leg, which forces the blood to travel via the side street collaterals instead of by way of the major arterial highway.

Opposite the arteries are the veins, thin-walled, low-pressure, low-resistance conduits that carry deoxygenated blood from our organs and tissues back to the heart, on the systemic side, while carrying oxygenated blood from the lungs back to the heart on the pulmonary side. Blockages of veins might cause no symptoms, minor pain, mild swelling of the affected organ, or severe swelling, and gangrene. Thrombosis of lower extremity veins is a common complication after any surgery and can lead to life-threatening pulmonary embolus. A great deal of time and money is spent trying to prevent this complication. Special stockings, foot and leg pumps, and anticoagulation are all in the armamentarium of deep venous thrombosis prophylaxis. I might be old-fashioned, but I still believe that a properly performed operation, coupled with early ambulation, is the best prevention. But, I still employ lower extremity sequential compression devices, a type of leg pump, on all my major operations.

Any obstruction to the normal flow of materials through our vast and complicated networks of biologic conduits disrupts the normal physiology of the human body. The surgeons of this world work diligently to keep our precious bodily fluids flowing freely, allowing the proper delivery of essential elements, and removing all the evil humors our bodies can produce.

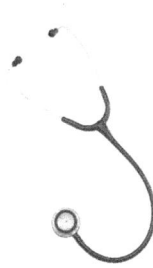

4. Leaks

"All bleeding stops...eventually"

~ Common OR principle

In many ways surgeons are akin to plumbers. If normal flow is disrupted, either blocked or leaking, we are both called out. And, like plumbers, sometimes the situation is an emergency, and sometimes it is a minor annoyance. Leaks in one of our human pipes or conduits can be a life-threatening emergency or a simple, self-sealing event without any significant consequences.

A ruptured Abdominal Aortic Aneurysm (AAA) and trauma to a major blood vessel are examples of major leaks that can cause sudden death. Surgeons are called in to rapidly diagnose the condition, direct replacement of the lost blood and fluid, and institute definitive intervention to repair the diseased or injured vessel. In such situations, the surgeon is called to repair the leak. Either by repairing or replacing the broken pipe; rerouting the normal flow around the leaking area, while closing off the leak; or permanently closing off the conduit, allowing the blood to flow through an alternate route or necessitating removal of the end organ.

Thus, a ruptured AAA almost always involves replacing the weakened aorta with an artificial graft. A tangential laceration to the inferior vena cava usually calls for direct repair. Bleeding from a femoral psuedoaneurysm, due to infection, calls for ligation, or tying off, the bleeding artery and rerouting the normal blood flow through a graft, taking a route away from and around the infected area. Bleeding from a splenic artery, lacerated by trauma suffered in a motor vehicle accident, will necessitate ligation of the artery and, most of the time, removal of the spleen.

At the other end of the spectrum, minor trauma to a leg might cause disruption of capillaries and small vessels in the skin and underlying tissues. Leakage of blood from these small vessels leads to swelling and pain in the area. As the pressure in the tissue rises and clotting mechanisms are activated, the injured blood vessels are sealed off, and the bleeding stops. The unfortunate, injured party has suffered a bruise. A collection of blood in the area is called a hematoma, which merely means swelling secondary to blood.

In between sudden death and minor bruising is bleeding; that is, at a slow enough rate to allow time for proper pre-operative evaluation, bleeding that might be contained within body cavities or closed spaces, and bleeding that is persistent, but at a rate that is not fast enough to be immediately life-threatening. It is the surgeon's job to treat each case on its own merits and decide which course of action is best.

A bleeding duodenal ulcer that requires surgery is often treated with suturing the vessel closed and then taking steps to prevent a recurrence in the future, a definitive anti-ulcer operation. Bleeding from a malignant tumor is best approached by removal of the tumor, ligating or tying off the leaking vessels in the process. Bleeding into the chest, around the lung, for whatever reason, is almost always treated, at least initially, by placing a tube into the pleural cavity, which is the space around the lung. The tube evacuates the blood and allows the lung to expand, thus tamponading (compressing) the source of bleeding and controlling the leak. This works best if the bleeding is from the low-pressure pulmonary circulation. Bleeding from systemic arteries in the chest, such as intercostals or bronchial arteries, will persist, and surgery will often be necessary

Why doesn't an injury to a major blood vessel, or for that matter, any blood vessel, always lead to uncontrolled bleeding and death? What is it that often allows the surgeon time to call in the OR crew? Our body has several mechanisms that protect us. First, and fortunately for us, there are blood clots; this clot formation seals injured vessels and halts the flow of blood. Our blood vessels also have the ability to constrict, decreasing flow, and facilitating clot formation. Sometimes all it takes is a properly directed finger, temporarily plugging the hole until definitive repair is possible. Over the years, I've had many patients that have been taken to surgery with an ER nurse holding direct pressure on a bleeding artery, being prepped into the field, until definitive control had been achieved.

Leaks that spring from arteries and veins are only one type of pipe surgeons are called on to repair. General surgeons, in particular, are frequently called to attend to perforations along the course of the GI tract. Such events are serious and life-threatening. Technically, the GI tract is outside of our bodies, a long tube that snakes its way from mouth to anus, bringing nutrients in and dumping unwanted waste out. A variety of digestive juices are dumped into this long tube along the way, while bacteria are also residents, aiding in the digestion and absorption of a variety of essential materials. These bacteria are welcome as long as they stay in their place. However, should our GI tract spring a leak, the digestive juices and bacteria can wreak havoc

Trauma, tumors, inflammatory conditions, ulcers, blockages, and many other disease states can lead to perforations and leakage of GI contents. Sometimes these holes are tiny, and our bodies have the capacity to seal them without surgical intervention. The "Watchdog" omentum is of great help when a leak pops up within the peritoneal cavity. Sometimes the hole is large, or the segment of the GI tract is very diseased, and a simple patch job won't suffice. In these cases, the diseased segment is best removed, or, if removal is not possible, then the GI contents are diverted away, either by creating an ostomy in a segment of bowel upstream from the damaged area or via an intestinal bypass of the diseased segment.

For example, Millie was an 88-year-old lady who came to the hospital, complaining of severe constipation, weight loss, and lower abdominal pain. Evaluation with history, physical exam, lab, and Computed Tomography (CT) scan of the abdomen and pelvis revealed a large tumor in her pelvis and free intraperitoneal air, suggesting that her intestine had perforated. She underwent surgery and was found to have a perforation of the colon, actually in the cecum, which is the beginning of the colon, which is where the appendix is located. She had a large tumor in the upper rectum which had caused obstruction of her colon, which had become extremely distended and eventually blew out, not at the point of obstruction, but at its weakest part, the cecum. The tumor in the rectum was growing into the surrounding pelvic organs as well as the left external iliac artery and vein, which made removal of that segment of rectum unsafe. The options at this point included simply repairing the perforation (not a wise choice); removing the perforated segment; reanastamosing the colon; repairing the perforation and creating a colostomy proximal to the area of the obstructing tumor; removing the perforated segment, reanastamosing the colon and creating a colostomy proximal to the area of obstruction; or removing the area of perforation, leaving no anastamosis and creating an ileostomy, which is an ostomy created using the end of the small intestine, rather than the colon.

So many choices—what's a surgeon to do? The answer is: look at the patient. What is the patient's overall condition? How does the cecum look? Is there much contamination by GI contents? Does the patient have underlying comorbidities, such as Diabetes or Congestive Heart Failure? After considering each factor, a decision is made. In this case, the portion of the colon was resected and an ileostomy created. The patient had been ill for some time; she had lost weight and appeared emaciated. The procedure that was performed left no intestinal repair or anastamosis to heal, limiting the risk of post-operative breakdown and leakage, which would cause severe sepsis and probably lead to Millie's demise. At the same time the leak was removed and the GI contents diverted away from the inciting blocked rectum. Would this always be the proper approach? Of course not; a different patient with fewer underlying medical problems would possibly allow for a more aggressive approach. The art of Surgery, like all medical specialties, calls for flexibility in decision-making, with each patient treated in a unique manner, and treatment plans tailored to an individual's particular needs.

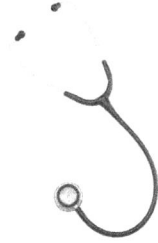

5. Stones

"The observer, when he seems to himself to be observing a stone, is really, if physics is to be believed, observing the effects of the stone upon himself."

~ Bertrand Russell

Stones come in a variety of shapes, sizes, and composition and can be found in a vast number of different locations. Some are valuable, such as gold or diamonds, but most are commonplace pebbles of no value. But, did you know that stones can be found inside our bodies? It's true; there are kidney stones, gallstones, salivary gland stones, appendiceal stones (appendicoliths), and a variety of others. They all have one thing in common: they serve no good purpose and, in the majority of cases, are the source of serious misery and sometimes life-threatening conditions.

Just why do all these stones form? There are numerous causes, such as inflammation, metabolic and endocrine abnormalities, reaction to foreign objects, or infection. Stones can be a simple annoyance, as was the case with my patient, Eloise, who complained that she had discomfort every time she sat down. My exam revealed a hard mass in her left gluteal area. She informed me that she had received an intramuscular injection in that area years before. Surgery was scheduled and what I found was, literally, a stone. Her body had reacted to that shot with an inflammatory reaction which, over the years, had become an irregular, calcified, hard mass: a stone. Every time she sat down she felt like she was sitting on a rock, because, every time she sat down, she *was* sitting on a rock. She felt much better after surgery, and her suffering was relieved.

Eloise was a simple case, and her surgery relieved a relatively minor irritation. What about more complicated stones?

The most common operation I do is cholecystectomy or removal of the gallbladder; as a matter of fact, this is the most common operation done in the United States. The majority of the time the patient undergoing surgery has gallstones. These stones can vary in size from grains of sand to tennis ball size (the largest I've seen, at least), and they can cause a variety of symptoms ranging from occasional episodes of pain to life-threatening sepsis to intestinal obstruction. Many people are walking around with gallstones who have never had a problem, but when they start causing symptoms, I've been told, that the pain is worse than being in labor.

Gallstones can obstruct the gallbladder, causing pain, either transiently or for hours or days; they can pass from the gallbladder, through the bile ducts and cause more severe pain; they can become lodged in the bile duct, causing obstruction which leads to jaundice and, sometimes, life-threatening pancreatitis or cholangitis; and, if a large gallstone makes its way out of the gallbladder and into the intestine, it can cause intestinal obstruction.

Cholangitis, or more properly, "ascending cholangitis," is a severe infection of the bile ducts that is often fatal if not treated expeditiously. Initiation of antibiotic therapy and emergent drainage of the biliary tree, either surgically, endoscopically, or radiologically, is necessary. Pancreatitis can be mild or life-threatening. Most cases of gallstone pancreatitis resolve over two or three days, after which cholecystectomy is usually performed.

Most of the time, problems related to gallstones are treated by simple cholecystectomy, usually laparoscopically, with tiny incisions. If stones in the main bile ducts are suspected before surgery, the patient is often evaluated with Magnetic Resonance Imaging (MRI) of the bile duct and, if stones are discovered, a friendly gastroenterologist can fish them out endoscopically before cholecystectomy is performed. This allows for complete treatment of the gallstones and their manifestations, with minimal discomfort or disability for the patient.

But, what if the stone or stones can't be removed? Suppose the stone is wedged inside a bile duct and won't budge. In such a situation, the art of surgery and the ingenuity of the surgeon come into play. Bile ducts, particularly, the major extrahepatic ducts, are vital structures; their purpose is to carry bile, which is produced in the liver, ultimately, to the intestine. This is an important excretory function and is important for the proper digestion of fats and the absorption of some vitamins. If the bile ducts become obstructed, the bile backs up, like a clogged sewer, and the patient becomes jaundiced. Stones and tumors are a common cause of biliary obstruction. Suppose the gastroenterologist has tried his endoscopic tricks and has failed. It becomes the surgeon's turn to step up to the plate.

Employing a variety of tools: choledochoscope, irrigation catheters, balloon-tipped catheters, stone forceps, and providence, the surgeon embarks on his quest to chase the elusive and, sometimes, stubborn stone. The gallbladder is rendered harmless first, either isolated or removed, and then the stone is approached. The first maneuver is to open up the common bile duct. It's very important to be sure that it is the bile duct and not some other structure. I usually will stick a small needle in and aspirate to be sure it's bile inside the duct and not blood. I know of at least one surgeon who opened the bile duct only to find out it was the portal vein; massive bleeding followed and the patient barely survived. Once the duct is open, the choledochoscope, a small fiber optic scope, is introduced; this allows direct visualization inside the bile ducts. Bear in mind that bile ducts are often small, usually 8-15 millimeters (mm) in diameter and sometimes smaller; they can only be safely opened so much, and there is always the potential for long-term sequelae if they are not treated with respect. The choledochoscope allows me to look up and down this narrow conduit and almost always shows me where the stones are. Often, the stream of saline that runs through the scope as I look, washes the stone free, and it is easily removed. Occasionally, the stone is stuck, wedged in position. My former boss, Dr. Dibenedetto, always said that it was biliary tract surgery that separated the men from the boys, and I have to agree with him; battling to free a large stone from the Common Hepatic Duct or from an area even more proximal can test the mettle of the finest surgeon.

I had a case recently that fit into this category. A young woman, Maria, presented to the ER complaining of abdominal pain and back pain. Tests revealed gallstones, and she was jaundiced, with a bilirubin level of about 5, normal being less than 1.0. An MRI confirmed Common Bile Duct Stones, and a gastroenterologist was consulted. He performed the expected Endoscopic Retrograde Cholangio-pancreatography (ERCP) and found stones in the Common Bile Duct and Right Hepatic Duct, which he could not remove endoscopically. The biliary system is rightly called the biliary tree, the branches forming a tree-like pattern. Imagine a tall, slender tree; the main trunk is the Common Bile Duct, the Gallbladder would be a large pouch attached to the trunk, the Common Hepatic duct would be just above this pouch, and the Left and Right Hepatic Ducts would be the first two big branches.

With the endoscopic approach being unsuccessful, surgery was the next step. The complexity of the situation did not lend itself to a laparoscopic approach; the surgery commenced with an old-fashioned right subcostal incision, which means a scalpel cuts about a six-inch opening paralleling the right lower ribs, the muscle is divided, and the abdominal cavity entered. First, the gallbladder was removed, and then the bile duct was approached. Working within my rules of surgery, the duct was first aspirated with a small needle, insuring that bile and not blood was flowing through the structure.

The duct was opened, and two stones immediately popped out. *Maybe this will be easy* was my first thought; it was also my last good thought for a while. The choledochosope was introduced and stones were seen in the common bile duct and in one of the more proximal ducts, presumably the right hepatic duct, as seen on the ERCP. The stones in the common bile duct were removed fairly expeditiously; utilizing a balloon-tipped catheter and irrigation, two additional stones were removed from this part of the bile duct.

The stones in the right hepatic duct were another story. One stone could be seen, but it wasn't budging. Stone forceps would not grab it, stone baskets were too small to snare it, and the balloon-tipped catheter broke. Even more frustrating was the fact that the stone could be palpated. Dissect a little higher and open the duct where the stone was sitting? There was a great deal of inflammation and swelling around the duct. Attempting such dissection could cause irreparable damage. Besides, the stone is *right there.*

Almost two hours later, little progress had been made.

There's an old saying, "I'd rather be lucky than good." Maybe the surgery gods finally took pity; whatever the reason, I stumbled upon the proper technique. With the balloon catheter behind the stone and with gentle traction, forceful irrigation was employed. This must have caused transient dilation of the duct, and the stone, with the traction from behind provided by the balloon, popped free, and it was quickly grabbed. Finally done, right? Wrong. Behind that stone was another one, also wedged in place. Fortunately, I had a technique that I thought would work. The next stone was removed in only a few minutes; however, there was a third stone lodged in the duct. This one actually came out with even less fuss. Finally, there were no more stones. A T-Tube was placed into the duct, which was closed, and the operation came to an end after more than three hours. Maria made an uneventful recovery.

Then there are rare times when the stones in the bile duct aren't even stones. Although it wasn't my case, during residency, my senior resident, along with the Chief of Surgery, was doing a common bile duct exploration and pulled a multitude of stones from the common duct. The stones were put into a container, but instead of just sitting there, the stones started to jump around. Perhaps you're thinking Mexican Jumping Beans; close, but not quite. Actually, the "stones" were *Clonorchis Sinensis,* a type of liver fluke. The patient had travelled years before in Asia and must have picked them up in that part of the world.

Challenging cases like these are relatively rare

these days. Most of the time, the offending common duct stones are removed endoscopically, prior to surgery, leaving the gallstones to be removed along with the gallbladder itself, utilizing minimally invasive laparoscopic techniques.

What about other stones? Urologists attack the problem of kidney stones on a regular basis. The stones they battle are usually smaller, but can be just as deadly and certainly painful. Kidney stones are usually composed of calcium compounded with other materials. These stones can, like gallstones, sit quiescent for years, silently, causing no problem. Large stones can form in the kidney and cause recurrent infections and, eventually, destroy that kidney's function. Smaller stones can pass from the kidney, through the ureter, and then out the bladder. Such passage results in excruciating pain, often with associated bleeding. Passage of the stone brings immediate relief.

Sometimes, however, the stone gets stuck in the ureter, blocking the flow of urine. The obstructed kidney continues to make urine, and the ureter and renal collecting system above the obstruction become dilated. Infection often follows and this can cause severe, life-threatening sepsis. Immediate intervention by the urologist then becomes necessary. Typically, this means passage of a stent to provide an avenue for the urine and treatment with antibiotics. Sometimes, the Urologist will remove the stone or pulverize it. Urologists, being much more creative and innovative than General Surgeons, have a vast arsenal of weapons at their disposal to bring to battle. Besides stents to relieve obstruction, there are also stone baskets, lasers, and extracorporeal lithotripsy. And, if all these tools fail, the friendly neighborhood Radiologist can be called to place a tube directly into the kidney, a nephrostomy, which allows the urine to drain while the Urologist plans another attack at a later date. Which particular approach is utilized depends on the exact location of the offending stone and the overall condition of the patient.

What about other stones? Salivary glands can form stones which obstruct the flow of saliva, leading to pain, swelling, and infection. Treatment is with antibiotics, then surgery to remove the offending stone.

Stones can form in the pancreas, usually a sign of long-standing, chronic pancreatitis and often a cause of severe abdominal pain that might be difficult to eliminate. Severe atherosclerosis, or hardening of the arteries, can be considered a type of stone that forms in the walls of our arteries. The normal, elastic arteries become rock-hard narrow conduits, altering or obstructing the normal flow of blood.

Stones composed of hardened fecal matter can form in the appendix. Such stones might just sit there, causing no particular problem or, probably more commonly, such stones block the appendiceal lumen and cause acute appendicitis. Appendicitis in this situation seems to differ from the appendicitis that is seen without these so-called appendicolith. The clinical course seems to progress rapidly, and perforation might occur in a much shorter period of time. One other consideration, particularly if the appendix has perforated, is to be sure this stone is removed. Such a stone would typically be a congealed mass of vegetable matter, bacteria, and calcium. Leaving it behind almost guarantees a post-operative infection.

Such a scenario played out in a patient of mine about twenty years ago. The patient, Augie, had undergone what had seemed to be a fairly routine open appendectomy. The appendix had been perforated, but infection had been localized to the area around the appendix. He seemed to be progressing well on the first post-operative day, but on the second day after surgery, he became sick. I found him cold and clammy, heart rate 135, blood pressure 90/50, and temperature 103. He complained of increased abdominal pain and was a bit more tender in the right lower quadrant of his abdomen, where his ruptured appendix had been sitting two days before.

I didn't think a CT scan was going to change my decision to re-explore Augie, and he was brought back to surgery. What do you think was found? An infected, inflammatory mass composed of small bowel, omentum, and pus and, in the middle of all this, a hard, 1.5 cm appendicolith which was removed with a few choice epithets, mostly aimed at myself. Augie's condition quickly improved after this surgery, and he was discharged home about a week later.

Such a case demonstrates that any surgery, even the most routine, carries the potential for severe, life-threatening complications and that stones inside of us are, almost universally, causes of misery.

6. - Oma

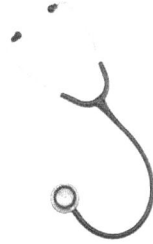

"Growth for the sake of growth is the ideology of the cancer cell."

~ Edward Abbey

"Oma" is a Latin suffix that means swelling. "Oma" is one of the most common reasons an individual might seek medical attention and end up in the OR. General surgeons deal with a vast array of "omas" every day. Lipomas, carcinomas, sarcomas, hematomas, seromas, and on and on.

On almost any day in my office, a patient will arrive with a complaint of a "lump on the arm" or "swelling on the back." The patient will say he has a cyst or was told he has a "lipoma." Lipoma is a fatty tumor; literally, fat swelling. These common, benign tumors can appear almost anywhere in the body—anywhere there is fat, that is. Most of the time, they are only a minor annoyance, causing a noticeable lump that is painless or causes mild discomfort. Most commonly, they appear just beneath the skin, little round balls that roll around, but I've also seen lipomas deep within muscles, growing behind abdominal organs, and in almost any body part one can imagine. Those that are superficial and symptomatic can often be removed in the office under local anesthesia. A small incision carried down to where the tumor sits, a couple of spreads of a clamp or scissors, and the ball of fat pops out. Over the years, I've seen a large number of patients whose bodies are covered with these annoying little lumps. Sometimes the patient requests that all of them be removed at the same time. The most I've ever removed at one sitting is 36, which required general anesthesia. Unfortunately, this same patient returned years later with about forty new ones. Another, similar patient just learned to live with them. He related how his father also had numerous lumps and had never complained; therefore, he had no reason to complain.

Sometimes one type of swelling can lead to another. Marvin was an elderly man who came to see me in the office, complaining of a lump on his side. My exam revealed a mobile, well-delineated mass on his right flank that had all the characteristics of a simple lipoma. I excised it in the office and sent him on his way. Two days later he called, complaining that the lump had returned. He came back, and it was obvious that he had bled into the site previously occupied by the lipoma. He now had a **hematoma**. I removed a couple of stitches and evacuated the blood and, once again, sent him on his merry way. Five days later he called again, saying that the lump had recurred. He returned to my office and, sure enough, there was swelling at the site of the original excision, but no sign of infection or bleeding. This time I stuck a needle in the area of swelling and drained off about 20 cc of thin pink fluid. The hematoma had now become a **seroma**, which means a swelling secondary to the accumulation of serous fluid. Serous fluid accumulates in any area of injury. Technically, it is blood devoid of most of the red blood cells and proteins that are normally in the bloodstream. Such fluid accumulates at the site of surgery after every operation and usually is reabsorbed by the body after a few days or weeks. But, back to poor Marvin. It was now more than a week since his lipoma had been removed and he still was plagued by a bothersome lump. After the fluid was drained with the needle, it recurred. At this point I drained it one more time, but also reassured Marvin that it would eventually go away completely. He returned a few weeks later for another check-up and, sure enough, the fluid was gone. Luckily, he never developed any infection, which would have required opening the wound, draining out the pus and, most likely, leaving it open to heal from the inside out, a sometimes drawn-out process.

Lipomas, hematomas and seromas are benign processes. Very often, lumps and bumps and swelling in various body parts are due to a far more ominous medical condition: Cancer.

The medical term for almost every type of cancer ends in the suffix "oma." Carcinomas arise from epithelial tissue. Thus, a squamous cell carcinoma arises from squamous epithelial cells, which are found primarily in the skin, lungs, esophagus, anus, and vagina. An adenocarcinoma is a cancer arising from tissue that normally forms glands; that is, the tissue secretes something. Adenocarcinoma of the pancreas refers to cancer arising from the glands of the pancreas. Adenocarcinoma of the lung arises from glands that lie along the pulmonary bronchi. Lymphomas are a different class of cancer; they develop in lymph nodes, small filter stations that are found throughout the body. These special immunologic strainers help remove infectious agents that are trying to invade the body, but they also remove tumor cells that are migrating from a primary tumor site. Lymph nodes can also be the site of primary cancers, lymphomas. Their role as filters also make lymph nodes a common first stopping point if a cancer should start to metastasize (spread).

Just about any tissue in the body can develop a cancer. The brain can develop gliomas, astrocytomas, or meningiomas. Bones can harbor osteosarcomas, which arise from bone cells, or medullary sarcomas, which arise within bone marrow. Kidneys can grow Renal Cell Carcinoma; the most common breast cancer is Infiltrating Duct Cell Carcinoma; lungs develop Bronchogenic Carcinoma, which can be adeno or squamous, but there are other types as well.

Volume after volume has been written about the various types of cancer; each type is its own disease. It can almost be said that every individual cancer is a unique disease, as those of us who intervene to try to stem a cancer's growth must tailor each treatment regimen to the individual patient.

For example, a breast cancer that is small in an elderly patient might be adequately treated by simply removing the mass and nothing else. At the other end of the spectrum, a breast cancer that has invaded the skin, spread to axillary lymph nodes or to distant organs in a 33-year-old woman requires aggressive treatment, combining chemotherapy, radiation, and surgery.

But, why do cancers behave the way they do? Why do some sit in one spot, nearly dormant, only to burst out after five years and rapidly invade their benevolent host, choking off the very source of their existence? Why do other cancers simply disappear, never to cause a moment's distress? And, why do some cancers grow and grow and grow, become unsightly, ugly, infected masses, but never leave the organ of origin, never spread through the blood stream or lymphatic vessels to lymph nodes or distant organs? All these questions are still being studied and, perhaps at some time in the future, a magic bullet will be discovered and any cancer that pops up can be discovered and eliminated at an early stage.

What is it about cancer that is so deadly? First, cancers can cause symptoms. A colon cancer in the sigmoid colon can grow to the point of causing obstruction, a surgical emergency. Cancers can bleed and cause severe anemia. That same colon cancer that is growing in the cecum (the first part of the large intestine) often will bleed small amounts of blood each day. Over time, anemia will develop and the individual might complain of feeling weak and tired or might pass out. The bleeding is not apparent because the small amount of blood that is lost is mixed into the stool. At the other end of the spectrum, cancers can erode into major blood vessels and cause spectacular and life-threatening hemorrhage that requires emergency intervention. A bronchial tumor that grows into an artery can suddenly start bleeding; the blood fills the bronchus and causes airway obstruction and coughing up of massive amounts of blood. If not controlled immediately, either by surgery or radiologic embolization of the offending artery, the patient can succumb in a very short time.

Some cancers cause almost no symptoms until it is too late. Pancreatic cancer is notorious for growing to a large size before it causes any symptoms. By the time it is discovered, it usually has grown into major blood vessels or other structures that make surgical removal impossible. Pancreatic tumors that are in the head of the pancreas, close to where the pancreas meets the intestine and bile duct, are more likely to cause symptoms when they are still small and possibly removable by surgery. Such tumors might cause obstruction of the bile duct, resulting in jaundice of the duodenum, resulting in intestinal obstruction.

In the final, late stages of cancer, the pathways all converge. The primary tumor has released its minions, who have settled in distant places: lung, liver, brain, almost any organ. These unwelcome invaders steal the life blood from normal tissues, impair normal organ function, cause pain and eventually death. It is the terminal cancer patient who led to the development of hospices. Hospices originally were real places, but now stand for more of an attitude; one that says death should come with dignity and should be pain free. Hospice care is truly a blessing to our patients in the terminal stages of their lives.

Discussion of all these different –omas could go on and on and on. Cancer is a word that strikes fear into most people, fear of the disfigurement that can come from the cancers growth or from its treatment, fear of the pain that can come from its presence, and fear of death. But, cancer, much of the time, is just another chronic disease, like diabetes or heart failure. Most of the time, it is controlled and its growth stopped or slowed, allowing the patient to live a normal productive life. However, like a sudden heart attack, which can take a life in moments, cancer can also progress rapidly, invade normal organs in a matter of days, and quickly cut down a promising life.

7. Foreigners

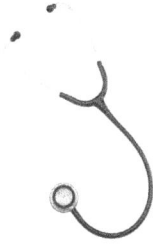

"Travelers never think that they are the foreigners."
~ Mason Cooley

One of the common tasks surgeons are called to perform is the implantation of foreign objects to reconstruct damaged areas or provide access to body systems to facilitate therapy. A variety of catheters (specialized tubes), meshes, artificial body parts, and stents are employed to replace old, worn out, damaged parts with shiny new ones.

Orthopedic Surgeons replace old, arthritic hips, knees, and shoulders with artificial prostheses that allow the patient to return to normal, productive lives. Cardiologists expand narrowed arteries with metal stents, allowing blood to flow normally. Urologists pass stents to allow urine to flow around blocked ureters. And, General Surgeons are called upon to place venous access catheters, which allow infusion of high calorie parenteral nutrition, administration of chemotherapeutic agents, and removal and replacement of circulating blood during dialysis. We also utilize a variety of prosthetic meshes to repair hernias or replace tissues that might have been lost to cancer, radiation therapy, infection, or injury. Artificial plastic grafts are often used to bypass blocked arteries or to provide access for dialysis.

All this implantation of foreign and artificial materials plays a vital role in maintaining the well-being of the sick and injured, relieving significant disability, and allowing these patients to live more normal lives.

But, what if something goes wrong? In general, our bodies would prefer that such foreigners remain foreign. In most circumstances, the human body responds to invasion by foreigners with an inflammatory response, trying to sequester and eliminate the invader. Infectious agents like bacteria and viruses usually cause us to feel ill, such a feeling telling us that something isn't right. An implanted piece of wood, no matter how sterile it might be, will pretty much always be rejected. Similarly, a sponge that is used in surgery and left behind will generate inflammation and, eventually, become infected, and also need to be removed. How is it that we are able to implant such a wide variety of foreign objects without suffering similar rejection?

The answer is in the materials that are used. Non-reactive metals and plastics are designed to generate minimal inflammation. Venous access catheters and artificial joints are examples of implanted objects that are designed to be tolerated by our bodies or ignored, as long as they do their job and aren't allowed to harbor any evil villains, such as bacteria. Should they, or for that matter, any foreign material, become infected, they almost always require removal, which means more surgery.

Mesh materials and vascular grafts are asked to behave in a bit of a different manner. Rather than be ignored, such implants are designed to become part of the family. Most meshes used for reconstruction are engineered to be incorporated into the body. The cells that are integral to the healing process insinuate themselves into the multitude of interstices of the mesh, collagen fibers grow into the mesh, and the mesh and the body work together to accomplish the task of providing structural support. Such meshes have tiny holes or grooves or pores to allow it to be integrated into the body system. Once again, infection with bacteria almost always requires removal.

Vascular grafts are usually composed of poly-tetraflourethylene (PTFE), which is the same material used in Gortex winter coats, or Dacron. Vascular grafts made from these materials are fashioned to allow bloodflow without thrombogenesis, that is, they won't clot off easily, while they become incorporated into the surrounding tissues. As blood flows through such grafts, a layer of cells grows on the inside of the graft, forming an endothelial lining, just as is found in normal arteries and veins.

But, what if these foreigners behave badly? What if all the good intentions go awry and these guests become a nightmare for their host? Infection, migration, rejection, and thrombosis; each of these can occur and cause our patients days, weeks, months, and, sometimes, years of misery. As previously stated, infected prosthetic material (artificial foreign objects) almost always require removal. Sometimes this is as simple as pulling out an infected catheter; but, just as often, a more invasive procedure is needed.

An infected vascular graft can cause local infection in the area where the graft sits, but by virtue of blood flowing through the area, can carry the infection almost anywhere in the body via what are called septic emboli. These are blood clots, usually small, that harbor the infecting bacteria. Depending on the location of the graft, such emboli can lodge in the legs, feet, brain, arms, fingers, or intra-abdominal organs, in short, anywhere. Removal of the graft is almost always mandatory. But then, what happens to the part of the body the graft was serving? What happens to the legs when an infected abdominal aortic graft is removed? Or to the abdominal viscera when a thoracic graft is infected? What if the infection has spread from the graft to the surrounding organs? Such cases are all potential disasters. Operations in such situations are designed to isolate the infection and replace the graft in a way that avoids the infected area, or, if necessary, to replace the graft after the infection has been eradicated

One example of the worst kind of disaster that can occur with graft infections is the case of Dennis. He was admitted to the hospital with fever and lower abdominal pain. He had a history of severe arterial occlusive disease and had undergone previous aorto-bifemoral bypass surgery, an operation to restore circulation beyond an occluded distal aorta and iliac arteries. A Y-shaped graft is utilized to bypass the blocked arteries. Dennis had previously had a portion of his graft removed because of infection and had undergone a high, above-knee amputation of his right leg and a left below-knee as a consequence. The concern with this admission was that the remainder of his graft, which had not been removed, was infected and the cause of his fever. While testing was being done, he developed upper GI bleeding, always a cause for worry, but more so in a patient with a known history of an infected aortic graft. The proximal parts of such grafts lie in juxtaposition to the duodenum and erosion into the duodenum, can cause a dreaded aortic-enteric fistula, a hole connecting the aorta to the duodenum. Such a fistula causes massive bleeding and requires emergency surgery. Dennis was diagnosed with just such a condition and was immediately taken to the OR.

At surgery, he had the expected hole in his duodenum, which was repaired and patched. The offending graft was removed with plans to simply repair his aorta. Plans sometimes go wrong, however. Dennis' aorta more or less fell apart. Simple repair was impossible. After considerable blood loss, the best that could be done was to ligate (tie off) the aorta just beyond the renal arteries, maintaining blood flow to his kidneys.

After surgery, Dennis, initially, was pretty stable. However, his fever returned and completion of the initial evaluation revealed that he had osteomyelitis of the pelvis and vertebral bones. It was likely that it was this infection that had extended to the aorta and his remaining graft and led to all his symptoms. It would be nice to say that Dennis' story ended on a happy note, but about three days post-surgery, he developed ischemic changes in his legs and buttocks, essentially the lower half of his body was dying due to lack of circulation. There was little to do short of what is called a hemicorpectomy, a controversial, disfiguring operation that would have removed everything from the waist down and left him with a colostomy, urostomy, and no legs or pelvis. No one could be found who would perform this procedure, and it was unlikely Dennis would have survived such a surgery. He passed away about two weeks after his surgery.

Infection is not the only mishap that can occur with these foreign materials. Implanted objects can become dislodged or migrate or otherwise move around to cause all manner of mayhem. Intravascular catheters sometimes break off and find their way into the heart of lungs where they can wreak havoc and usually have to be fished out by our friendly interventional Radiologist.

Years ago there was a device called an Anglechik prosthesis. This was a donut shaped plastic device that was used to prevent gastroesophageal reflux. The donut was wrapped around the esophagus at its junction with the stomach and was supposed to be a mechanical barrier preventing reflux of gastric acid up into the esophagus. I never had the opportunity to deploy one, but the surgical literature reports that the Anglechik didn't like to stay in its intended position. Apparently it used to migrate all over the place, and there were frequent reports of it being passed through the GI tract and out via the colon and rectum. No one is quite sure how it made its way *into* the GI tract in the first place.

Rejected foreigners are a much different story. Sometimes it seems like the body can cast these materials out. Bullets often are lodged deep inside body cavities, but, over the years, it is common for our body to reject their presence, and gradually bring them to the surface so that they can be easily plucked out by some intrepid intern. Joe comes into the office complaining of a lump in his leg. He reports that he was shot ten years before and the bullet was never removed. Somehow, over time, that bullet, which had been lodged deep in the muscle of the thigh, has been pushed out into the subcutaneous tissue. Sometimes it starts to erode through the skin, but it is usually removed under local anesthesia in the office, plucked out, and cast into the requisite metal pan with a resounding clang.

Of course, bullets and metal pans have to go together. Every movie and TV show that depicts a bullet being removed always includes that "*clang.*" One time, as a second-year resident, I was assisting an intern who was removing a bullet from a patient's back. As she neared completion, I noticed that there was only a plastic basin on the field. I immediately instructed her to stop what she was doing and asked the circulator to get a metal pan. The intern looked a bit confused as I remained silent until the proper equipment was available. Once the pan arrived, I allowed her to proceed. She cast the bullet into the pan with a "clang" that was worthy of the best western. She thanked me later.

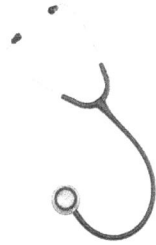

8. Forces

"There are only two forces in the world, the sword and the spirit. In the long run the sword will always be conquered by the spirit."

~ Napoleon Bonaparte

A significant portion of training in General Surgery involves the management of trauma. Trauma is caused by the application of external force to an individual, resulting in an injury. Thus, trauma can be as minor as a paper cut or as major as the injuries suffered in an explosion.

Starting with a paper cut: the edge of a sheet of paper, oriented appropriately and drawn across the skin with sufficient force, penetrates the skin and causes a painful, superficial cut in the skin, usually through the epidermal layer and into the dermis. Bleeding ensues, which can seem profuse. In a normal individual, such an injury is a minor annoyance, treated with a band aid. However, just like in a well-known television advertisement, even such a minor event can cause significant bleeding in someone with hemophilia or some other bleeding disorder.

A paper cut is an example of what is classified as penetrating trauma. The force is applied through an object to a concentrated area, causing damage only to those areas that directly contact the object. More well-known causes of penetrating trauma are stab wounds and gunshot wounds. These weapons cause greater injury by imparting greater force, but still over a relatively small area. The sharp blade of a knife, combined with the attacking force of an assailant, can cause severe injury and death. A razor sharp sword would be expected to cause greater harm than a kitchen knife, but even the simple kitchen knife wielded in the proper manner, with sufficient force, can cause serious injury. Like the paper cut, but on a larger scale, the force applied to the knife is transmitted to the victim via the blade. A narrower, sharper blade imparts its force over a smaller area, creating more injury, but to a smaller area than a larger blade. A stiletto type knife causes injury via its sharp point. A switchblade is more suited to a slashing type assault, but, with a sharpened tip, can also penetrate quite effectively.

Bullets carry much larger force and initially might impart damage to a small area. However, as a bullet penetrates, the large force is transmitted to the surrounding tissue, leading to severe injury. Bullets often ricochet off structures, creating even greater damage. Shotguns fire a large number of pellets that initially are tightly packed. As they travel through the air, these pellets are scattered, and their kinetic energy is dissipated. At close range, shotguns can cause massive trauma as the pellets become dispersed within the target tissue and organs. A shotgun blast at close range might cause a fairly small entrance wound, but the exit wound usually is considerably larger, and the swath of damaged tissue can be enormous.

The results of these penetrating forces range from minor scrapes and lacerations to death. A knife plunged into the abdomen cuts through skin, fat, muscle, peritoneum, and any organs in its path. Massive contamination from injured bowels, bleeding from severed arteries and veins, and neurologic injury from cut nerves all can result from a single violent in-and-out thrust. The surgeon's job is to resuscitate the injured party, diagnose and treat the injuries, and then see the patient through to recovery. Resuscitation is done in accordance with the ABCs of trauma: Airway, Breathing, and Circulation. Diagnosis might be as simple as examining the patient, seeing bowel hanging out through the stab wound, and deciding to go the OR. However, diagnosis might be more involved if the extent of the penetration is not readily apparent. In this age of widely available CT scanners that are running 24 hours a day, such imaging provides a wealth of information as the tract of the knife often can be clearly seen on modern CT scans, and details of the injuries might be obvious on the images obtained.

At the other end of the trauma spectrum is what's called "blunt trauma," with motor vehicle accidents being the most common type. Blunt trauma delivers its forces over much larger areas, often to the whole body. Persons who jump from tall buildings, trying to imitate birds, will invariably plummet to the ground and suffer injury secondary to the sudden impact with the ground. The rapid deceleration can transmit great force, breaking bones, tearing solid organs, blowing out lungs, shearing spinal cords, and causing brains to bounce around inside their hard, encasing skull.

The forces applied often seem to me to be greatest in one area, particularly in motor vehicle accidents. I don't think this has ever been studied closely, but if the legs have suffered a very severe injury, other parts of the body will often have relatively minor trauma. Of course, it is extremely unfortunate if the greatest force is delivered to the head, shearing it off, a scenario I've seen at least once. The blunt, so-called "multiple" trauma patient who arrives in the Emergency Department always demands a thorough evaluation. In this age of rapid evaluation via CT scanner, this routinely includes scans of the head, neck, chest, abdomen, and pelvis. There is still a role for plain X-rays of the extremities.

What about devastating, combined, blunt, and penetrating trauma? Blast injuries, common in war zones, can cause blunt trauma by the rapidly expanding gases of a blast or sudden impact of the victim thrown by the blast, penetrating injury by shrapnel that is propelled into the victim, and burn injury from the heat generated by the blast. The great forces involved can be enough to completely disintegrate the injured party, leaving nothing behind.

The most devastating injury I ever saw was a patient, Michael, who had been in a boating explosion. He suffered burns about his face, neck, and shoulders from the blast, multiple rib fractures, and bilateral pneumothoraces (collapsed lungs), a lacerated liver, bilateral fractures of the tibia and fibula, aspiration of salt water, and hypothermia from immersion in the waters of the Long Island Sound. He was awake and alert, however, and he did survive after being treated with endotracheal intubation, bilateral chest tube placement, fixation of the orthopedic injuries, watchful waiting for his liver injury, skin grafts to his head and neck burns, prolonged ventilator support, treatment for pneumonia, tracheostomy, and a few months of rehabilitation.

Such a patient demonstrates the incredible resiliency we humans possess. We can be beaten, broken, slashed, burned, shot, stabbed, and blown up, and, amazingly, bounce back completely. Truly amazing.

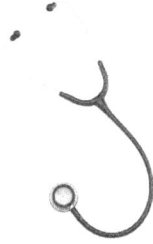

9. Fixing a Hole

"Probably the closest things to perfection are the huge absolutely empty holes that astronomers have recently discovered in space. If there's nothing there, how can anything go wrong?"

~ Richard Brautigan

One of the tasks surgeons are often called to perform is to fill in holes. A hole is defined as an opening through something or a cavity within a solid object. If our body develops a hole, it's usually not a good thing. Defects created by disease or, sometimes, by treatment, need to be corrected.

Cancer therapy, be it surgery or radiation therapy, can leave a void that requires reconstruction. Sometimes, this can be as simple as bringing adjacent tissues into play and closing an open wound, as is done after mastectomy for breast cancer. Other times, a Plastic Surgeon might be called upon to transfer tissue from a distant part of the body into the defect, so-called pedicled flaps or free flaps. Surgical research and anatomy have been able to demonstrate that certain muscles or combinations of muscle and skin can be raised from their usual anatomical site and rotated or stretched to fill in holes some distance away.

The head and neck defect created by radical surgery for cancer can often be effectively filled in by flap, utilizing the *pectoralis major* muscle. Breasts are often reconstructed using a TRAM flap, composed of abdominal wall muscle and skin. Patients get a bonus with this flap because it also includes a free tummy tuck.

Open wounds that are less complex are often managed with skin grafts. A thin sheet of skin of appropriate size is laid over a clean, well-vascularized wound, which then, like a newly sodded lawn, grows into the wound bed, allowing permanent wound coverage. Grafts can be full thickness of skin or partial thickness, depending on the wound's size and location. Areas that are subject to greater pressure or stress, like the soles of the feet, require full thickness, while areas which bear less weight can be managed with partial thickness grafts.

Some open wounds are managed merely by trying to create the proper environment within the wound to promote healing. Maintaining a clean wound, keeping bacteria levels low within the wound, and eliminating dead tissue all help to promote ingrowth of new tissue and eventual wound closure. Such healing, by what is termed "secondary intention," occurs over several weeks to months, but often is the best and safest option to fill in the hole.

Holes pop up almost anywhere in the body. In General Surgery, we're often called upon to fix defects in the abdominal wall, the famous hernia of song and story. Hernias can occur almost anywhere on the torso. Hernias in the groin, inguinal hernias, are most common; femoral hernias are also considered groin hernias, but are less prevalent. But, there are also lumbar hernias, obturator hernias, diaphragmatic hernias, hiatal hernias, incisional hernias, ventral hernias, and Spigelian hernias. All are characterized by weakness of the abdominal wall muscular or enveloping fascia which is designed to keep the abdominal viscera confined to its proper place.

Such defects allow organs to escape the usually friendly confines of the abdominal cavity, sometimes to commit great mayhem. In the old days, before elective repair of most groin hernias was recommended, hernia was the most common cause of intestinal obstruction. However, this is no longer true, having been supplanted by peritoneal adhesions, which usually are the sequelae of previous abdominal surgery.

For our patients, hernias appear as a bulge that can be felt beneath the skin. Most of the time, there is very little pain. The bulge, under the influence of gravity, becomes most apparent when the individual stands up and often disappears when reclined. The size of the herniated mass ranges from pea size to larger than a medicine ball. One of the most remarkable things about hernias is the sheer volume of abdominal viscera that manages to escape through what is often a relatively small hole in the abdominal wall. A patient might come to the office and complain of a mass that is 15 cm in diameter (about 6 inches). However, when examined, the hole in the abdominal wall might be only about 3 cm. It is truly amazing that so much bowel can pass through such a small hole and cause no, or very minimal, symptoms. It is true, however, that sometimes obstruction can occur, and these situations are true emergencies.

Bowels that herniate through abdominal wall defects can become trapped; incarcerated is the medical term. This incarcerated bowel becomes obstructed and can become strangulated, which means that the blood supply to that segment of intestine is cut off, and the bowel begins to die. Obstruction and strangulation are life-threatening conditions and require prompt attention, either manual reduction of the herniated intestine, which means to push it back into the abdomen where it belongs, or surgical repair. Even if the incarcerated bowel can be freed by reducing it back into the peritoneal cavity, repair still is recommended, to avoid repetition of such a serious, life-threatening complication of hernia.

The art of hernia repair has evolved considerably over the thirty years I have been in medicine. Medical school taught repairs that merely pulled the edges of the hole together; elaborate mesh repairs were reserved for the rare patient who had loss of tissue such that the hole could not be breeched by the patient's native tissue.

Inguinal hernias have been attacked via the Bassini repair, the McVay repair, the Shouldice repair, the preperitoneal repair and now a variety of mesh repairs. Bassini, McVay, Shouldice, and preperitoneal are very effective techniques, but each suffers from the property that dooms so many hernia repairs to inevitable failure, the old surgical demon: tension.

Hernias can develop for a variety of reasons, but one of the most common contributors to hernia development, and certainly to hernia enlargement, is tension. The groin, particularly in men, is a naturally weak area. There is only a thin fibrous sheath that prevents herniation, the *transversalis fascia*. There is a shutter mechanism which the body employs to add strength to the groin area. Specifically, when an individual strains, the abdominal muscles descend into the groin and act like a shutter to prevent bulging through the *transversalis fascia* that lines the floor of the inguinal canal. However, once this *transversalis fascia* stretches and weakens, the shutter mechanism is lost; each time the individual strains, the tissue is stretched a bit more, and eventually it weakens enough that intra-abdominal organs start to push through the floor of the inguinal canal, with the resultant direct hernia.

Modern repair techniques employ a mesh screen, which replaces the thinned-out weakened tissue with something strong. There are numerous options for mesh repairs, probably each as good as the next, as long as they are utilized in the appropriate manner. As in any operation, clean dissection, adequate hemostasis, and tension-free repair will result in excellent long-term results, no matter what type of mesh is employed.

One of the principles of mesh repairs is that the mesh itself not be subject to too much tension. The greatest stress on the mesh is at the edges where the mesh is usually fixed to healthy tissue by sutures or tacks or a combination. Mesh that is too small and only extends to the edge of the defect will allow the greatest stress at the weakest point and almost always leads to recurrence of the hernia. Most repairs now employ larger meshes that distribute the tension over a larger area and, thus, are less likely to recur.

There are other holes that occur in our bodies, defects that result from trauma, infection, and other disease conditions. One thing that is certain is that if a serious hole develops, it is a surgeon who will be called in to make repairs.

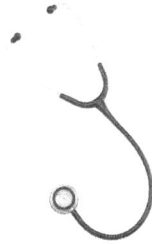

10. Treat the Patient

"The art of medicine consists of amusing the patient while nature cures the disease." - Voltaire

It happened again. A phone call from an Emergency Center at 2:00 a.m. requesting that a patient be admitted to my service. The ER physician explained that the patient had a small bowel obstruction, a problem commonly managed by general surgeons. I pressed the ER doctor for more history.

The patient was 31 years old, and had been sick for about twelve hours with abdominal pain, nausea, vomiting, and diarrhea. The obligatory abdominal and pelvic CT scan had been performed, and the reading was "small bowel obstruction." I asked for even more details, which was almost like pulling teeth. The patient had not had previous surgery, there were no apparent hernias on exam, but the CT report was unequivocal: "dilated proximal small bowel with collapsed ileum and normal appearing colon," the classic radiologic appearance of a small bowel obstruction.

I explained to the calling physician that, almost certainly, this patient did not have a small bowel obstruction; most likely it was acute gastroenteritis, and it would likely resolve spontaneously within 24 hours. The ER doctor persisted, however, stating that the patient had an elevated White Blood Cell (WBC) count at 21,000, there were ketones in his urine, and the Blood Urea Nitrogen (BUN) was elevated at 28. I did agree with his diagnosis of dehydration and that the patient would benefit from admission, so that intravenous (IV) fluids could be administered.

I saw this patient in the morning. His pain was gone, his nausea and vomiting had resolved, although he still had some diarrhea; the WBC count had decreased to 12,000, and the BUN was normal. I started him on a liquid diet, which he tolerated without problem, and he was discharged that day without any significant sequelae. In retrospect, the patient could just as easily have been managed in the ER with an infusion of IV fluids and discharged home with medication to address his symptoms, with admission being reserved only if he did not improve with such measures.

The scenario above is played out on an almost daily basis around the country. A patient is admitted to the hospital because an X-Ray or lab test suggests a certain diagnosis, even if a patient's clinical presentation suggests something completely different. The patient above gave a pretty good history for acute gastroenteritis. It is unusual for patients without hernias or previous surgery to develop small bowel obstruction, certainly not impossible, but definitely out of the ordinary. But, the hallmark of diagnosing intestinal obstruction is the X-Ray findings. The CT scan clearly demonstrated the classic appearance of small bowel obstruction. Sometimes, I wonder.

The clinical presentation of acute gastroenteritis is, typically, sudden onset of abdominal pain, often with cramps, nausea, vomiting, malaise, fever, and diarrhea. But, what happens to the bowel in such a situation? Does it become hyperactive, trying to expel some offending agent? Does it stop altogether and dilate, as our body's defenses are mobilized to attack the noxious invader causing the illness? Does the bowel contract, dilate, or does it do both? Perhaps the stomach dilates, while the small bowel contracts, or vice versa. I don't know. I don't think anyone really knows.

Common teaching about acute gastroenteritis is that it is an exclusionary diagnosis based on clinical presentation and the absence of any other discernible underlying cause of the associated symptoms. General consensus is that viral infection is the etiology, and it is a self-limited disease, usually resolving in two to three days. There have not been any good studies, at least to my knowledge, that document the CT scan findings of a patient suffering from acute gastroenteritis.

These days it seems to be common practice, by some physicians at least, to treat patients solely on the X-Ray and lab findings, often ignoring the fact that there is a patient attached to those images and numbers. These doctors are guilty of ignoring clinical judgment, treating the X-Ray, and not treating the patient. In my mind, it is one of the cardinal sins of modern medicine.

Diagnosis and therapeutic management of a patient requires that every aspect of the patient be included in the evaluation: history, physical exam, laboratory data, and imaging. Each factor is weighed against a variety of possibilities and a diagnosis is made. As I've written previously, (see Talking to Patients, July 10, 2010, *heardintheor.blogspot.com*), the majority of patients will tell you what is wrong within the context of a five- to ten-minute interview. All the testing that follows confirms or rules out the various conditions that appear within the differential diagnosis. The knowledge necessary to ask the proper, probing question is taught in medical school, and the skill is refined during residency and post-residency practice. In our modern, harried, defensive, get 'em in and get 'em out quick, medical world, taking the few minutes necessary to properly interview the patient might not be deemed as cost effective as ordering a CT scan.

And, if the patient winds up being treated for the wrong condition, well, the CT scan said they had it, and that's documentation enough to provide proper coverage of one's derriere.

The only problem with this approach is that the patient suffers. Far too often, patients are sent home because the WBC count or CT scan is normal, or admitted to the hospital because one or another exam is abnormal. The history and physical exam might suggest a serious condition, but the imaging and lab were unremarkable. Would it be better to forego such testing and base everything on clinical impression? Certainly not. As I've stated previously, it is best to approach patient care utilizing all the tools available. CT scans provide a great deal of information, including detailed images that help clarify a murky clinical situation and allow physicians to say it's OK to defer surgery or, conversely, to say that surgery is absolutely necessary.

For example, a 20-year-old male is minding his own business, sitting on his porch and reading his Bible, when "two dudes" come out of nowhere and shoot this poor, unfortunate soul in the right flank. He walks into the ER complaining of pain at the site of the wounds. There are entry and exit wounds, one just medial to the right anterior axillary line and the other posterior and a bit more lateral. The physical exam is equivocal and the chest X-Ray is normal. What should be done? In this case, the CT scan provides a wealth of information. Very often the latest model scanners will provide images that demonstrate the path of the bullet and provide information regarding damage to organs in that path.

I cared for a patient with this exact scenario recently. The path of the bullet was obvious, there was an injury to the right lateral aspect of the liver, and the bullet appeared to have nicked the right kidney. The only thing I couldn't be sure about was the hepatic flexure of the colon, a devastating injury if left untreated. I decided it would be best to operate on this patient. At surgery, the findings correlated perfectly with the scan. The bullet had travelled through the liver, just missed the colon and nicked the upper pole of the right kidney. The injuries required no special repair, just leaving a drain in the area of injury, and the patient recovered uneventfully.

What about a much different, but very common presentation? A few weeks ago, I was asked to admit a 10-year-old boy who presented with complaints of right lower quadrant abdominal pain, present for twelve hours. CT scan was done and reported as acute appendicitis. Specifically, the appendix was described as having enhancement of its wall, a sign of inflammation, and was minimally dilated to 7 mm, with inflammatory changes surrounding it. The boy was admitted to the hospital and seen by me about four hours later. When I evaluated him, he reported that the pain had disappeared. His exam was perfectly normal; by normal, I mean I could push on his abdomen through to his back and all he did was smile at me. What to do? In this case, nothing. I observed the patient in the hospital for about 8 hours more and then sent him home with instructions to his mother to call if any symptoms recur. Most likely, he had a self-limiting stomach bug that had caused the CT scan changes.

I suppose there are some surgeons who would have operated on that patient and, perhaps the appendix even would have been abnormal when examined by the pathologist. I have to believe, however, that it is always best to remember that radiologic images are only shadows, lab results are mere numbers, and there is a live patient who comes with both.

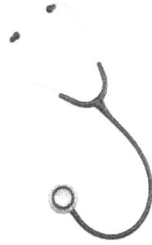

11. Things that are Heard

"It is the province of knowledge to speak, and it is the privilege of wisdom to listen."

~ Oliver Wendell

Over all the years I've been practicing surgery, I have heard patients tell me a lot of unusual and, sometimes, bizarre stories. Sometimes it's a simple thing, like an allergy; sometimes it's a totally implausible explanation for an unusual, and usually embarrassing occurrence; and sometimes, it's just funny.

When a patient comes to see me or is admitted to the hospital, one of the most important questions that is asked is, "Are you allergic to anything, particularly medications?" The answers are occasionally improbable and imaginative. Here is a list of some of the items patients have said they're allergic to and what the effect is:

Epinenephrine/Adrenalin (Given as part of CPR/Advanced Cardiac Life Support): "Makes my heart race; makes my blood pressure go up, made my heart stop."

Saline (typically used in IV fluids): "Makes me swell; made me short of breath."

Hydrocortisone (a hormone made by our adrenal glands): "Makes me swell."

Benadryl: "Makes me sleepy."

Anesthesia: "Makes me really sleepy."

Penicillin: "I've never had it, but my mother is allergic, so I must be, too." "Isn't everyone allergic to penicillin?" and "I developed a fever when they gave it to me."

Oxygen: "Caused a rash on my face." Turns out it was the plastic in the mask that was being used to administer the oxygen.

I'm sure there are others, but these are the most common. What is often ascribed to allergy is merely an effect of the medicine or treatment. Epinephrine stimulates the heart and is a mainstay of cardiac resuscitation. It has the effect of raising heart rate and blood pressure.

Saline is a small amount of salt mixed with water to create a solution that is close to the concentration found in our body fluids. Initially, the administered saline circulates within our blood stream, but after a while it will leave the circulating blood and diffuse into the tissue outside our blood stream. This causes these tissues to swell and occurs in everyone who receives significant volumes of IV fluids. If the fluid builds up in the lungs it can cause shortness of breath until our body eliminates it, usually via the urinary tract.

Hydrocortisone is made by our adrenal glands and is necessary for a large number of cellular functions. Hydrocortisone, or one of its synthetic cousins, is often used to treat severe inflammation, but has a side effect of causing swelling (among others).

Benadryl and anesthesia; no comment is needed.

Penicillin and antibiotics related to penicillin that employ a beta lactam component are often cited as a being "an allergen." When first developed, penicillin was less than pure, and these impurities often caused a reaction. Even so, many people are truly allergic to penicillin and related compounds. A rash, watery eyes, and difficulty breathing or throat swelling are hallmarks of a true allergy. If a patient describes such symptoms, then proper precaution is necessary.

What else do patients say? In the process of taking a patient history, particularly if surgery is contemplated, questions about bleeding tendencies are asked. I have been told on more than one occasion and usually without prompting: "I'm a semi free bleeder," almost always worded exactly like that.

The first time I heard this phrase, I was surprised and I queried further. Usually it means that the patient had excessive bleeding during some previous surgery, and the surgeon, rather than blaming himself for failing to secure adequate hemostasis, tells the patient that he or she must be a free bleeder. Never mind that all subsequent coagulation testing is normal. The reason it's "semi" is the patient has almost always had other surgery that has been uneventful, or is it that the "free bleeding" is only partial; that is, eventually the bleeding stops? (Of course, one of the maxims of surgery is that all bleeding stops...eventually.)

I've also learned that there are different levels of "free bleeding." Some patients describe themselves as pure "free bleeders"; others fit into the aforementioned category of "semi free bleeders"; then there are the lower level "borderline free bleeders"; and finally, what I assume to be the lowest level, the "borderline semi free bleeder." I'm really not quite sure what the exact order should be, and I'm not sure what modifications are needed to my surgical technique to compensate for these disorders. More research is obviously necessary.

The truly amazing thing is that over the years I have heard these exact phrases at least a dozen times.

"I was told I would die if I had this surgery." I hear this phrase or something similar about half a dozen times a year. It is usually uttered by a patient who:

1. Has significant comorbidities making any surgery high risk, usually of cardiac, hepatic, pulmonary or immunologic origin. Patients with such disease might have serious complications with any surgery, and no procedure should be undertaken lightly. However, in the face of life-threatening conditions, there is often little choice. Gangrenous or perforated bowels, necrotizing soft tissue infections, or open fractures, left untreated often have a mortality of 100 %. In such situations surgeons are forced to bite the bullet and proceed with surgery, offering some hope for recovery, but often after a stormy post-operative course.

There are other conditions that can only be treated with surgery. Ruptured AAAs are 100% fatal without surgical intervention. But, there is an ethical consideration. It is common for patients with known AAAs associated with severe pulmonary or cardiac disease to be advised to not have elective repair. The risk of death from the elective surgery is weighed against the risk of death from rupture, and a recommendation is made. It is likely, however, that somewhere down the road, rupture will occur and about half of the time the patient will survive to make it to the hospital. What to do? Previously the patient elected to forego surgery as too risky. Now, with the AAA having burst, the patient will undoubtedly die if nothing is done. Most of the time surgery is attempted, sometimes successfully, sometimes not. The significant underlying illness usually means a very prolonged recovery and, commonly, the patient makes it out of the OR, only to succumb days or weeks later, usually the result of progressive organ failure.

Should the surgery not be offered? If possible, all the potential implications should be discussed with the patient and/or family. Almost always they elect to proceed with surgery and hope for the best. In this day and age, we have not started rationing healthcare, but if restrictions on healthcare arise in the future, I suspect that such a scenario will play out far differently.

2. Has a surgical problem that might be difficult to repair or has a high potential for complications. Surgeons, being at least partly human, like to see their patients recover after surgery, with good outcomes. Hernias should not recur, arterial reconstructions should remain patent, and so on. There are patients who have conditions that make a successful outcome problematic. One example is very large abdominal wall hernias that have been left untreated for a prolonged period of time. Hernia is a defect in the abdominal wall that allows the abdominal viscera to migrate out of its normal position, into the subcutaneous tissue. In some cases, the majority of the abdominal organs are within the hernia, and a situation called "loss of the right of domain" exists.

This means that the space normally occupied by the bowels is gone, with the peritoneal cavity having contracted down to accommodate the smaller volume of contained viscera. In such a situation, it becomes very difficult to return the wayward bowels to their rightful home and position. Certain steps can be taken to facilitate the surgery: pre-op bowel cleansing, to insure the bowel is collapsed, prolonged pre-op nasogastric drainage for similar reasons, use of a "silo" system to slowly return the bowel to a gradually expanded peritoneal cavity, often employed in neonates with similar conditions (called omphalocele or gastroschisis). In any event, the patient with such a hernia presents a difficult problem and, rather than try to take the time to explain the condition, some surgeons will dismiss the patient by saying, "You'll die if you have this surgery so learn to live with it." I can never say this to a patient, because I don't know. I can explain that the surgery will be difficult, with increased risk for complication, death being included, but I have rarely categorically stated that a patient will die from a certain procedure. I have to say, however, that I have encountered patients who were so ill, with severe coagulation disorders or greatly weakened immune systems or overwhelming multi-organ dysfunction, that any attempt at surgery would be doomed not only to failure, but would likely hasten the patient's demise.

3. Has no or bad insurance. It is sad that in this day and age this issue arises, but unfortunately, it does. Some surgeons might refuse to attempt an operation because the patient has Medicaid or no insurance. Patients who are admitted to the hospital with surgical conditions, such as cholecystitis, most often are treated with the indicated surgery during that hospital stay. Some surgeons, after noting a lack of financial resources, will find a reason to not operate, and discharge the patient. These patients invariably show up in an ER somewhere else where another surgeon will do what's right and take proper care of the patient.

Physicians are called upon to treat the sick and injured. Nowhere does it say only the well-insured or wealthy sick and injured. Telling the patient that they "will die" if they have surgery does them a great disservice. Sadly, I've encountered dozens of patients over the years who have been told those exact words. It is remarkable how their surgical risk improves as soon as soon as they are found to have some financial resources.

Sometimes patients arrive in the ER with conditions that are "embarrassing." One that is commonly encountered by me, along with other general surgeons, is rectal foreign bodies. Vibrators, often still running; a variety of fruits and vegetables, most commonly cucumbers and potatoes; shampoo and soap bottles; flashlights, and almost any other object that can fit, have all been removed over the years.

Removing the object sometimes is as simple as

grabbing hold and pulling. More often it requires a little ingenuity. It sometimes seems like the rectum is holding on to the object with all its might, and of course, these objects never seem to have convenient handles that one can easily grasp. Then, there is the problem of getting one's hand into such a tight space. My hands are big enough to palm a basketball; it is almost impossible for me to get my whole hand inside, which means I'm usually trying to get the job done with three or four fingers.

I rarely ask the patients how the offending object made its way inside; the explanation is obvious. Nevertheless, the sheepish patient often feels compelled to offer an explanation:

"I accidently sat on it; I didn't know it was on the chair." I suppose the patient makes a habit of going around his home pantsless.

"My son was playing with it in the shower and I didn't know he left it there. I slipped and it got stuck." Do you always let your son play with a vibrator in the shower?

"I was trying to soften it up before I cooked it." (referring to a potato). I don't think I want to eat at your house.

"I was minding my own business when three guys shoved it in me."

"I guess it got loose and crawled inside." (referring to a hamster). Call PETA.

"I was massaging my prostate." Somewhat believable.

"I came home drunk, passed out on the bed, and my wife was so angry about my being drunk again that she shoved her vibrator up my butt and just left it there." Even more believable.

"It was a stupid thing." Definitely true in all cases.

The potential complications of such foreign bodies can be serious. They are often lodged in such a way as to put considerable pressure on the rectal or colonic wall, which could lead to perforation; or they might have sharp portions protruding, which can also cause perforation. They can also cause obstruction. If the object cannot be removed transanally, then exploratory laparotomy becomes necessary. This might require opening the colon to remove the object and might necessitate a colostomy. It is, therefore, in the patient's best interest to make every effort to remove the object transanally. Sometimes, I wish the manufacturers made the grips of these things with sandpaper built in; it would make things so much easier.

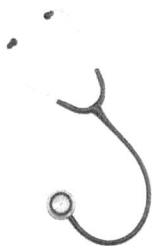

12. Seeing is Believing

"Always wear clean underwear in case you get hit by a bus and have to go to the hospital."

~ Mom

"The doctors are far too busy to notice if your underwear is clean or even if you're wearing underwear at all."

~ Dear Abby

Mom was right. In the course of caring for our patients, it is usually necessary that the patient disrobe at some point. In the case of emergencies, particularly trauma, the clothes are removed by the emergency staff, often by cutting the clothes away. This is a necessary part of the evaluation and treatment of our patients. Signs of injury need to be determined and the entire body requires examination.

I am telling you right now—no, warning you, dear reader—that everything is noticed. What is worn, contents of pockets, quality, quantity and presence or absence of undergarments; everything is noted by the treating staff. It is almost impossible not to notice;

sometimes such information might be helpful in the evaluation of comatose, unresponsive patients. Sometimes it provides a bit of a chuckle in an otherwise stressful situation.

The severely injured patient is resuscitated and evaluated in a fairly standardized fashion. Clothes, which stand between the treating staff and the injured party, are cut away, and the ABCs of trauma are followed as the patient is stabilized and evaluated. The staff in attendance includes the trauma surgeon, nurses, respiratory therapist, radiology technician, anesthetist, more nurses, surgical residents, and anyone else that is needed to adequately care for the patient. Although the greatest attention is paid to signs of injury, the staff is still human and not blind. Provocative attire, piercings, tattoos, and everything else is noted and comments are frequent.

The things we see are frequently unusual. Leopard skin thongs, meshed crotchless underwear, or no undergarments are common. Dirty underwear is also common. The population that suffers serious trauma includes persons who frequently overindulge in alcoholic beverages, illicit drugs, or a combination of both. Very often this class of individual pays little attention to their sartorial presentation. Commonly, the cleanliness of the undergarments correlates well with the number of teeth that are missing.

Moving on; tattoos are all the rage these days. Once limited to soldiers and circus performers, body art has moved into the mainstream, and some of these adornments are quite intricate and impressive. Some, on the other hand, are crass and tacky. Often hidden in the most private parts, tattoos can display attitude, send a message, or simply adorn.

The message, "No rear entry," with an arrow pointing down and stamped across the lower back clearly informs potential suitors of limitations that help to direct any amorous advances to appropriate venues.

"Sweet" tattooed on the left breast and "Sour" tattooed on the right sends a message with a bit of whimsy, although I doubt that there was truth in advertising.

Tattoos are often casualties of surgery. Incisions are placed wherever necessary to perform the operation in a proper manner. This might mean slicing through a tattoo or removing a portion. One poor naked lady tattoo suffered a mastectomy as part of her owner's femoral tibial bypass surgery. I've always tried to reconstruct this artwork as best I could and most of the time have done quite well. But, sometimes severely ill or injured patients need very expeditious surgery, and their body art suffers.

Piercings through every body part imaginable are also common. Breast, nipple, penile, vulvar, and clitoral rings are displayed to treating physicians on a regular basis. Patients reluctantly remove these adornments for surgery, but it is often necessary for safety reasons, depending on the surgery to be performed. One lady years ago absolutely refused to remove the clitoral ring she had worn for five years, even though she presented with an infection in her groin that was probably related to this particular body jewelry. I can only speculate on what that ring did for her.

Tattoos, piercings, and undergarments are intentional embellishments that convey a message, or provide a sense of well-being, personal pleasure or pride. But, what about the unintentional?

Belly buttons are a frequent focus of surgery in this age of laparoscopy that commonly starts with an incision in or around the umbilicus (belly button). Surgeons frequently comment on the cleanliness of their patients' belly buttons and the things that are pulled out sometimes are amazing. Lint by the bushel, waxy brownish material, crumbs of pretzels, bits of Cheetohs, cupcakes or cookies are pulled, scooped, extracted and otherwise removed from innies and outies prior to gallbladder surgery, appendectomies, and so many other common operations. Other unusual items are eraser heads, dead flies, beetles, and even a thumbtack. Grandma should have said, "Clean your navel in case you get hit by a bus and have to go the hospital."

Any body orifice or skin fold can be the resting place for unusual objects and buried treasure. One of my associates once lifted a lady's ample breast prior to beginning an abdominal operation and found a half-eaten sandwich. When queried later, she recalled that she had put it there, planning to finish eating it later and must have forgotten about it. Foreign objects frequently lodge in the esophagus, usually poorly chewed meat or something similar. Children are experts at swallowing, inhaling, and otherwise instilling coins, toys, rocks, and any other appropriately-sized object. Surgeons, Pulmonary, and

Gastroenterology doctors are often called to address such problems. Sometimes watchful waiting is all that is needed, but often the object requires removal. Over the years I've removed such mundane items as an open safety pin from the larynx, a mass of dried fruit from the small bowel, and Barbie's shoe from the right mainstem bronchus. Most of these procedures were years ago. Nowadays, I usually defer to my more specialized colleagues and allow them to intervene. The rectum is also a resting place for items of surprising diversity, but this is discussed more thoroughly in the chapter, "The Things That are Heard".

Ears are another site where unusual objects often find a resting place. For some reason, bugs tend to rest in the ears of young boys. Although I don't look in too many ears these days, in past years, I frequently was treated to the sight of flies, mosquitos, a praying mantis, beetles, and a variety of other creepy crawlies staring at me through an otoscope from the recesses of a small boy's ear. Taking these beasts out sometimes presented a bit of a challenge. The combination of an insect that often disintegrated into pieces and a screaming child made it easy for me to decide that my Ear, Nose, and Throat (ENT) colleagues were best equipped and trained to do such delicate extractions.

Looking back at my forty years in the medical world, I wish that I had kept all the things that I've fished out of patients and photographed some of the more bizarre sightings. Such things would have made for a very compelling museum of medical oddities.

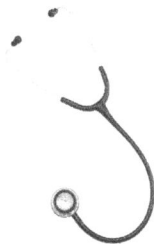

13. They Did What?

"There is a theory which states that if ever for any reason anyone discovers what exactly the Universe is for and why it is here it will instantly disappear and be replaced by something even more bizarre and inexplicable. There is another that states that this has already happened."

~ Douglas Adams

Over the years, I've been witness to a variety of actions done by patients, usually to themselves, that can be called unusual, baffling, bizarre, or worse. Attempts at self-treatment and self-enhancement often end up with tragic consequences. Patients who are ill sometimes do things that they would never do when well, actions that are often upsetting to their families or other patients.

When someone becomes ill, whether from severe infection, trauma, heart failure, or any other serious condition, the brain might behave in a less than normal manner. Metabolic changes caused by illness, the effects of medications, sleep deprivation, or altered perfusion secondary to shock can all cause patients to see things that aren't there, do things that are peculiar, or be certain that they are at their Aunt Minnie's home instead of in the hospital.

For example, many years ago, I had a patient named William who was in the hospital for a hernia repair. He was 88 years old. The evening after surgery, he resolutely got up out of bed, stark naked, went into the room next to his, and relieved himself in his neighbors waste basket. He then nonchalantly returned to his room and went back to sleep. The lady in the room next door was a bit upset, but no harm was really done, and the next day William had no recollection of the event. Perhaps he had been sleepwalking, or perhaps it was the influence of the pain medication he had received.

Elderly people becoming confused for a period of time after major surgery is very common. Over the years, I've seen this happen dozens of times. Families often become upset if Grandpa doesn't seem to know them or thinks they're still 12 years old, but it is almost always a transient phenomenon. Of course, the doctors involved always search for a reversible cause, doing their best to be sure the patient is not hypoxic (low oxygen levels), septic (severe infection), in heart failure, or anything else. Once satisfied that no unexpected complications are about to rear their ugly heads, the family is reassured that it is most likely a combination of the effects of anesthesia and post-operative medications that are making their loved one confused and that he will, most likely, be back to his old self in a few days. In my experience, it takes about four to five days, but I've seen it take as long as four months for an elderly patient to completely return to their baseline condition. One caveat, patients with Alzheimer's disease almost always regress somewhat after illness that requires major surgery, and some never return to the previous level of cognition, which is sad.

Patients who are sick often need to have catheters, IV fluids, and drains invading their bodies. Patients who are sick also are often confused. Very often these two things don't go very well together. It is not uncommon to make rounds and find a patient holding their nasogastric tube, central IV line, drainage tube, or urinary catheter in their hand, sometimes looking confused, but just as often looking triumphant. I don't know what goes on in the minds of these ill patients, but I suppose it is not surprising for a little voice to say that they're not supposed to have a tube going down their nose into their stomach or another one going up into the bladder. Sometimes these unexpected decannulations are only a nuisance, requiring simple replacement of the tube, but sometimes it can lead to a major setback.

Endotracheal tubes, which go through the mouth or nose into the trachea, are used to provide for mechanical ventilation. Some patients are so sick that even being off the ventilator for a few minutes can be life-threatening. Foley catheters are occasionally pulled out by patients. Such catheters have a balloon on the end and if pulled out with the balloon inflated, serious bleeding can occur in males, the aptly termed "balloon prostatectomy." The bleeding can be profuse, but, thankfully, usually stops spontaneously. Finally, there are surgical drains. Major operations often require leaving a drainage tube in the area of the operation to allow the removal of blood; or anticipate leakage of bodily fluids, bile or GI contents; or allow decompression of structures while healing occurs, such as with a T-tube after bile duct surgery. If such a drain is removed prematurely, replacing it is usually not possible without a return to the OR or intervention by a radiologist. Such procedures always carry the risk of complication.

In the world of drains or tubes, surgeons learn to anticipate such events. Important drainage tubes are sutured in place, often with two stitches and dressed in an inconspicuous manner so that the patient remains as unaware of its presence as possible. Patients sometimes need restraints or sedation, particularly those on mechanical ventilators, to prevent self extubation. There are very few things as uncomfortable as having a large tube passing down your throat and into your windpipe. I'm sure it makes you feel like you are suffocating, while it is actually helping you survive. It is in the patient's best interest to prevent them from pulling such tubes out.

Patients sometimes undergo procedures that set them up to take a fall. Diabetic patients and patients with peripheral vascular disease often end up with amputations, be it part of the foot, below the knee, above the knee or at the hip. At some point during the post-operative recovery period, be it at two weeks or two months, these patients forget that they are missing part of their leg. They get up from a nap, or in the middle of the night, and try to walk. It is actually not that surprising. After amputation, the nerves which have been divided apparently are unaware that the foot or leg is missing. They send signals back to the brain conveying information that the body is still whole; thus, the aptly named phenomenon of "phantom pain," or pain felt in a foot that is no longer there. Along the same lines, a patient, especially one who might be half asleep, gets up to go to the bathroom, "forgetting" that their leg is now in the Pathology department. Frantic calls in the middle of the night from family members are common, usually relating that Grandma fell; she forgot she didn't have her right foot anymore. Sometimes their wounds get torn open, and patch jobs are required. Some patients say they still have the feeling that their leg is there, even years after amputation.

Sometimes our patients are just lucky. They do something that should cause great harm or even death, but they come through completely unscathed. As a resident on the Trauma service, we had a patient, Carlos, who had suffered a closed head injury. He was in this country illegally, having come from El Salvador. For the better part of six months, he was in the hospital, 14/15 on the Glasgow Coma Scale. This means that he was nearly normal; all he lacked was comprehension. He spent all his days on a special bed designed to prevent bed sores called a Clinitron bed. He received physical therapy on that bed, he ate on that bed; I don't think he left that bed for all the time I was involved in his care.

Well, one day he must have decided to try to

escape the confines of that accursed bed by eating his way out of it. I have to explain that a Clinitron bed is designed to put very little pressure on any part of the body. It is essentially a big balloon filled with sand that is circulated by a blower inside. This creates a buoyancy that keeps the patient on the surface of the canvas balloon. When Carlos chewed through the canvas balloon the sand began to blow around him, gradually burying him. He was found completely covered in sand with only his mouth and nose sticking out. Another inch of sand and he would have suffocated. God looks out for fools and children.

Patients with altered mental status as a result of disease or injury are only one subgroup of patients who sometimes do things that are out of the ordinary. Surgeons frequently are called to see patients who have attempted to treat themselves, sometimes with disastrous results.

Self-improvement is one area where people sometimes act without truly considering the consequences. Attempts to enhance certain body parts is one area where physicians sometimes have to shake their heads and wonder, "what was he thinking?" One intrepid young man got the bright idea that he could enlarge his penis in the same way women enlarge their breasts. He had read of silicone injections and decided that if it was acceptable for women then it certainly should be adequate for men. Direct injection of silicone long ago was replaced by implants for breast augmentation. Nevertheless, this young man logically concluded that injection of silicone into his penis would make this organ larger and, therefore, make him more desirable. Medical grade silicone was probably not readily available and, besides, the stuff at the local Home Depot was surely just as good. He bought some silicone caulk and proceeded to inject it into the shaft of his penis. To make a long story short, he didn't succeed in making a short penis long. Instead, he turned his private part into a hard, irregular lump that required several surgeries by the Urology service to be returned to some semblance of a normal organ. It never again functioned properly, working only as a conduit for urine, but good for nothing else.

Cancer is a scary word for almost all of our patients. Images of major surgery causing permanent scarring and deformity, and weeks or months of chemotherapy and/or radiation therapy with concomitant side effects pop into the mind when the "Big C" is mentioned. Most patients accept the treatment which has actually become far less disfiguring, with fewer side effects in recent years. But, there are patients who insist on treating this disease in their own way.

I saw a patient, Meg, several years ago, with breast cancer. About one year before she saw me, another surgeon had removed a lump from her right breast which was an infiltrating duct cell carcinoma, the most common type of breast cancer. Further surgery was recommended to insure that there was no residual cancer and that there had not been any spread to other parts of the body. The patient and her husband refused, electing to treat this disease with high doses of carrot juice. I'm not sure exactly how much carrot juice they drank, but when they came to see me, both were bright orange.

I examined Meg and found she had a recurrent mass in the right breast, in the same area her previous cancer had occupied. She did allow me to do a needle biopsy at that time, which confirmed that her breast cancer had, as one would expect, recurred at the site of the previous excision. A segmental mastectomy and axillary lymph node dissection was recommended (this was in the days before sentinel node biopsy). Initially she agreed, but, she and her husband talked it over, and she changed her mind and decided to continue the carrot juice regimen, doubling the dose. Despite all my efforts, she left, didn't return any calls, and I didn't see her again for about a year.

This time she was in the hospital with widespread metastatic disease. She did agree to chemotherapy at this time, but her response was not very dramatic, and she eventually succumbed to her disease. Carrot juice does have some benefits. It is high in beta carotene, which is an antioxidant and does provide health benefit. However, intoxicating your body with carrot juice is a very poor method of controlling cancer. Of course, it could be true that she would have responded just as poorly to conventional treatment, but I doubt it. Her initial mass was less than 2 cm with no sign of spread. With proper therapy, there was a very high chance she would have been cured.

There are large numbers of patients who come to be seen only after "doctoring" themselves has failed. Surgeons see a large number of patients with cutaneous abscesses these days, most caused by resistant Staph Aureus. Treatment involves a combination of antibiotics and drainage of the abscess. Patients commonly tell me that they've had similar problems previously, but usually took care of it themselves. This usually was done with some type of drainage, often with a kitchen or pocket knife, warm soaks in Epsom Salts, heating pads, or over-the-counter (OTC) ointments and salves.

Surprisingly, such home remedies are often successful, but occasionally home remedies can lead to worse problems. Ginny was such a case. She started with an abscess on her abdomen. She convinced her son to open it up, which he did with his pocket knife (cleaned with alcohol first). Initially all went well; she felt better and the abscess seemed to improve. However, the abscess was in her lower abdomen, beneath the area that was usually obscured by her big belly. For whatever reason, a nasty infection developed where the abscess had been, caused by a combination of bacteria. It spread very quickly and she became very ill. She was brought in to the hospital by ambulance with a blood pressure of 60/0. She had developed a necrotizing infection in her abdominal wall. She was taken to surgery expeditiously and had all the necrotic tissue removed. Five operations and four weeks later, she left the hospital, a lucky survivor. She did, however, lose fifty pounds in the process, down to a svelte 240. Still, it was a very tough way to diet.

Sometimes we see patients who have not been thinking clearly, whether it be from mental illness or intoxication, and decide to perform surgery on themselves. Years ago, a patient was admitted to the trauma service after stabbing himself in the abdomen. He was evaluated by locally exploring the wound, which went through the abdominal wall muscles. The decision was made to explore his abdomen; the surgery was to be performed by one of my co-chief residents. He found that the knife had penetrated down to the peritoneum, but did not pierce this layer. Consequently, there was no serious injury, he was closed up, and he had an uneventful post-operative course. He was cleared by the Psychiatry service and discharged home. Two weeks later he returned with his abdominal wound open and bowel hanging out through the opening. It turned out that he had stabbed himself in the abdomen again. He went back to surgery and, once again, it was found that the knife had penetrated to the peritoneum, but not through. It was far enough to cut the suture that was holding him together, however. After this surgery he was asked why he did it and how he knew to stop before the peritoneal cavity was violated. His answer:

"At night I start drinking, and then I get depressed. That big knife looks like a good way out, if you know what I mean. But, as I stab myself it really starts to hurt and I stop."

The very sensitive peritoneal lining saved him. As aforementioned...God looks out for fools and babies.

Finally, there are the professional patients, people who, for one reason or another, find ways to be admitted to the hospital. Why should anyone want to spend their days in the hospital? Many reasons. The professional patient might be homeless, seeking drugs, trying to get a respite from incarceration, or might really be sick.

One patient who was well known up and down the Texas coast was Charles. He was in and out of hospitals from Corpus Christi to Dallas, almost always with an abscess in his thigh. I first saw Charles in one hospital with a different diagnosis: subclavian vein thrombosis. He had been in hospitals so frequently that he almost always needed central venous catheters to administer the necessary IV antibiotics. One of these central lines probably caused the blood clot; the treatment was anticoagulation with heparin and then Coumadin. I didn't think twice about Charles until the next time I saw him with an abscess in his thigh. He had several previous drainage procedures, and I did another. He healed fairly rapidly and was discharged, his parting words were that his girlfriend would stop by my office to pay his bill. I didn't hold my breath and, of course, the mythical girlfriend never appeared. Well, Charles kept showing up at different hospitals, always with a new abscess in his thigh which required drainage and antibiotics. While in the hospital, he would zip up and down the hospital corridors in his wheelchair, go down to the patio to smoke and visit with other patients, and, in general, have a grand old time with three square meals a day, nurses waiting on him, and never a worry about anything. I don't know where he went upon discharge, but after a short time, he'd show up at another hospital with a new abscess. He was well known in ERs all over the city.

My last encounter with him was years ago. He was admitted with an abscess in his thigh (what a surprise) which required drainage in the OR. The abscess was beneath the fascia in the lateral right thigh and grew a pure culture of yeast, which is a bit unusual. I was pretty sure he had injected his thigh with something to cause such an abscess to form. Rather than confront him, I took a different approach. I asked him if he wanted to get better; he replied in the affirmative. I then informed him that the way to eradicate his infection once and for all was for him to stay in bed with his leg elevated. I instructed the nurses to take away his wheelchair, and I ordered strict bed rest. This meant no smoking, no patio, and no schmoozing with other patients. I don't really know if I succeeded in curing him, because I received an angry call from this disgruntled patient. I went to see him and told him that everything I'd ordered was necessary for him to heal adequately. He responded by firing me, certainly not unexpected. From that day forward, whenever he showed up in the ER, and I was on call, I would respond to the call from the ER physician by informing him that Charles had fired me in the past and had said he did not want me involved in his care and that they'd have to find another surgeon. He was last seen in one of the local hospitals many years ago. I have no idea what became of him.

Other patients have tried other things to force their way into the hospital. One lady said she'd had massive upper GI bleeding and produced a bag filled with bloody fluid. She kept reporting vomiting blood, always disappearing into the bathroom and emerging with a basin filled with bloody emesis. After several days, the nurses discovered a large bottle of ketchup she'd hidden in her purse. There was a similar patient, only he took it a step further. He would suck on his IV tubing and fill his mouth with blood and then expel it into a basin. It was only when a nurse went to check on him in the bathroom when he was "retching" that his *modus operandi* was uncovered. As a resident, we had a patient who was in the County Lock-up, which was conveniently located behind the hospital. This patient had an above-knee amputation which had recurrent infections. All the residents knew that he smeared stool in the open wounds, keeping them infected. On his last admission, we cleaned up the infection, healed his wounds, and then put his amputation stump in a cast, shielding it from any tampering. He went back to jail in this cast, with plans that he follow up in our clinic in about one week's time. However, he was transferred to an upstate prison only a few days later, and I never saw him or his stump again.

Finally, there was Martha. She came to the ER complaining of severe pain in her groin and bleeding from her vagina. The ER physician had evaluated her with a pelvic CT scan which revealed an inflammatory process in the area adjacent to her rectum and vagina. At about 2:00 a.m. I came to see her. She was tender in the right groin, and the CT revealed this pocket of gas and inflammation to the right of her rectum. She would not allow a rectal exam, claiming she was too tender. The CT revealed bulging into her rectum and I made the diagnosis of a supralevator abscess, which is treated by drainage through the rectum. At surgery, I found the area that was bulging into her rectum, tried aspirating with a needle and then opened it up. A small amount of fluid drained out, but there was no severe infection. Additionally, I found the source of her vaginal bleeding: a small puncture wound in her vagina, which was actively bleeding. I had very strong suspicions that she had injected something through the wall of her vagina. Her family later reported finding bloody gloves and syringes in the garbage at her home. After surgery she was very demanding. I did my best to tend to her needs, asked the psychiatric service to evaluate her, and, once I was sure that any infection had been adequately treated, she was discharged, never coming back to see me.

There are many other examples of misguided patients doing things that make me and other physicians scratch our heads in wonder. In the end, however, the whys don't matter; we take care of the acute problem, address underlying issues as well as we can, and realize that there are social ills we can't do anything to cure.

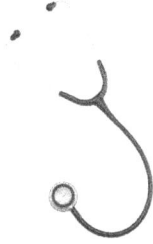

14. On the Fringe

"All action takes place, so to speak, in a kind of twilight, which like a fog or moonlight, often tends to make things seem grotesque and larger than they really are."

~ Karl von Clausewitz

*O*h...no...SCREECH...CLANG... and, then, a shower of broken glass. *What happened? I can't feel my arms. Is that my blood...someone help me...someone help...*

"Shine that light in here...quick...he looks pretty bad...at least he's still breathing. "

"Thank God, just look at this car, we're going to have to cut him out. Hey buddy, can you hear me?"

I open my eyes and try to smile. There's an ache in my chest and I can't feel my legs.

"Just relax, buddy, we'll have you out in no time."

The noise of men working, cutting the mangled car away from me, fills my ears and, finally, arms wrapped around my chest and legs; hands on either side of my head, and I'm gently pulled from my brand new Ford, only had it for two weeks. I'm glad Lilly and Jess weren't with me.

What's this on my face, I can't breathe; take it off.

"Relax, Mr. Jameson, it's just oxygen. Let's go…God look at those legs. Let's move it."

I look up into his eyes and see only determination as I'm rolled over a few bumps and loaded into the back of the ambulance. A loud siren sounds as I sense the ambulance racing away.

"Let's get some IV access. What's his pressure?"

"Got a 16 in this arm, Ringer's is running wide open…pressure's 70/30, heart rate 120. Hang on, Joe, we'll be there in five minutes."

I guess they found my wallet. I hope they're calling Lilly.

"County, this is 190, we've got an MVA, auto vs. truck, single casualty, male, 35 years old, facial trauma, possible left pneumothorax, bilateral tib fib fractures, Vital signs, sinus rhythm 120, last BP 70/30, O2 sat 99 on 100% face mask, positive LOC. ETA three minutes."

"Don't worry, Joe, the trauma team at County is the best. You stay with me."

I try to smile, but it hurts to move my mouth.

"That's OK, here's the hospital. Let's go, everybody."

A silent, bumpy ride carried me into the hospital ER. A bright light shined from the ceiling; *not the bright white light,* then, from every direction, masked and gowned people descended, the sound of cutting as my bloody clothes are cut away.

"Can you hear me, Joe?" asks a disembodied voice,

but I can't respond.

"Heart rate's 140, BP 70, no breath sounds on the left, we need a left chest tube, airways OK, for now, O2 sat's 98."

I feel a cold splash on the left side of my chest, a short needle prick, and then a sharp pain in my chest.

"Heart rate's still 140, BP 80...he's not responding to us... go ahead and intubate."

Something hard and cold is put in my mouth and I tighten up and try to scream as a plastic tube is shoved down my throat. *I can't breathe...I can't...*but then I pass out completely.

"Are you there? Open your eyes. That's better. You're looking better..."

"There's a lot of blood, probably two liters...that spleen looks like hamburger; no way to save it...there's a hole in the diaphragm...he'll need a chest tube..."

I think I'm supposed to be asleep or maybe I'm just dreaming all this. I can't feel a thing at least. This sounds like a new voice...

"Those legs look pretty bad; bones are pretty smashed. At least the nerves and blood supply seem OK. Let's just wash both wounds out and put him in an external fixator for now. How's he doing? We'll try to be quick..."

My whole body feels numb; from the neck down there's nothing. Maybe I'll try to move...Yeow...not a good idea. Pain from my chest to my toes.

"Are you having pain?"

Dumb question. I've got a tube in my throat and something in my nose and shoved up my private parts. At the moment my chest, stomach, and legs feel like someone has been pounding them with a sledge hammer.

"Nod your head if you are having pain."

OK, I'll nod my head, if that will make you get up off your ass and do something.

"I'll get you something right away...here comes your doctor."

I can't hear you guys, but I'll bet you're talking about me. What's happened to me? I know I was driving along and then there was this big truck, and I guess it hit me.

"Joe, can you hear me? Good. I'm Dr. Sunny. You were in a pretty bad accident; ruptured your spleen, tore your diaphragm, broke a bunch of ribs, broke both legs. You've got a breathing tube in right now and a machine is breathing for you. Are you having any pain? Squeeze my hand if you're in pain."

I give him a real tight squeeze.

"OK, I get the picture; nothing's wrong with your grip, I see. We'll get you something right away. Take a deep breath for me...Good...and another...very good. You're doing very well, I think. I hope we'll be able to get some of these tubes out soon. I'll check on you later."

I hope that nurse gets back soon. Finally, I hope this pain med works...quickly...

It's dark outside, I wonder what time it is, hell, I wonder what day it is. No more numb feeling; less pain in my abdomen, but my legs hurt more. Just relax...be patient...this can't go on forever.

"Oh, you're up, that's good. I need to turn you, but, don't worry, we'll be as gentle as we can be and it's bath time, give us a chance to look at your back side. Rachel, can you give me a hand with Joseph? Everything's looking good, Joe. Vital signs are normal, O2 sat 100%, good urine output, you're moving everything; I think the worst is over."

She's a nice nurse; I certainly hope she's right. I don't like this tube in my throat. What are you doing...gentle...gentle with these turns...those legs are broken. That bath feels good...keep going ladies...don't stop now...careful on the legs. Well done, I feel much better.

I was able to relax for a while after this. The nurse came in and checked on me regularly, and she was pretty good; gave me the pain med regularly without asking, turned me as gently as possible and even took time out from her busy schedule to just hold my hand for few minutes. I felt a bit guilty that I didn't remember her name, even though she had told me at the beginning of her shift. I did learn the next day that she was Maggie. I don't remember her as being the greatest looker, but she was a sweet soul and, from my point of view, completely dedicated to the well-being of her patients. I remember this conversation.

"Dr. Smoot, Joseph here needs better IV access. Look at his arms, all blown up and he's been stuck a million times," she said to one of my doctors, although I don't recall any Dr. Smoots. Must have been a resident.

"That peripheral looks OK to me, Miss Hatch."

"It's only a 22 and it's been in for three days. If it blows I don't want to stick him a dozen times. He's still got a chest tube on the left. Can't you just pop in a central line; only take you a few minutes. The big game doesn't start for at least thirty more minutes."

"OK, OK, get everything ready, and I'll be back in ten minutes."

He really was pretty slick putting in that line. He really did just pop it in; only took five minutes, and it made my life a lot easier. Finally, some sense of peace.

Something's wrong. I can't breathe. My chest feels like there's a gorilla sitting on it and pounding it with his fists. I can't breathe...I can't...

Fog, all there is...I open my eyes and all I see is fog, I can't feel anything, I can't see anything, are my legs there, are my arms there? Nothing but fog.

I'm not sure how long it took for the fog to lift. It was like a part of my life was gone. I learned later that it was almost two weeks. One day I opened my eyes and I saw Maggie looking at me. I could feel my arms and legs, and there no longer was a tube in my throat. The tube was now going through my neck. There was a small tube in my nose and my stomach felt full.

"You really gave us a scare, Joe. You had pretty bad lungs, but now they're better. Oh, don't try to talk. They had to do a tracheostomy, but it should be more comfortable for you without that tube going through your mouth. Before you know it, that tube will be out, and we can finally have a real conversation. Oh, and they had to put a new tube in your gallbladder. But, don't worry; I've seen much sicker men pull through and you're definitely on the mend."

How about one of your special baths, dear Maggie?

"Oh, and give me a few minutes and I'll be back to

give you your bath. That's what I like to see, a smile. I'll be back in five minutes."

It was a fine way to emerge from that fog. After the bath came physical therapy; even though it hurt a bit, it really felt good to get my arms and legs moving. The next day, they took the tube out of my nose and I actually got to drink something. My chest felt better, and I was able to breathe without the machine.

"Hello, Joe. It's good to see you on the mend. It's Dr. Sunny. I'm going to switch that trach tube. It'll just take a second and then you'll be able to talk."

I grabbed his arm as he reached for the tube and stared into his eyes.

"Don't worry, Joe. I've done this a hundred times. You'll be able to talk, be able to swallow a little easier, and in a few days, you won't need any tube at all. I can tell you haven't lost that strong grip you had when we first met. Just relax and I'll be done in no time."

He was right; it didn't hurt, and I could talk with that new tube. My voice was a bit raspy, but I did have a voice. The following day, I moved to a different room, out of the ICU and away from Maggie and all the other nurses who had helped me through my ordeal. My legs were on the mend and they got me up, first just sitting, then standing, and finally, I took some steps. Baby steps, but to me I felt like I'd just finished a marathon. After that I recovered my strength fairly quickly. I was moved to the Rehab unit for a couple of weeks and, after forty two days in the hospital, I walked out. I actually was wheeled to the door, but I insisted on walking from the exit door to the car that was waiting.

I later learned that the driver of the truck that hit me had been drinking and talking on his phone. He apparently didn't fare as well. He smashed into his windshield and died instantly. I saw the pictures of my new car and could barely recognize that it used to be a car. I look up at the sky frequently now, looking towards Heaven and thanking whatever might be up there for giving me back my life and for nurses like Maggie, doctors like Dr. Sunny, and for all the other nurses, doctors, therapists, technicians, aides, and everyone else who help people like me, day after day and night after night.

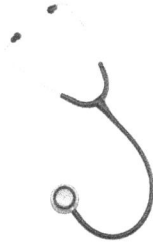

15. Dinnertime

"Eating is not a crime. It's not a moral issue. It's normal. It's enjoyable. It just is."

~ Carrie Arnold

Lorraine ate today, and it was a moment worthy of celebration. Two months ago she was in surgery having a dead segment of colon removed. Now, after ventilators, dialysis, and multiple trips back and forth to the OR, she is able to eat. And it's not just tolerating tube feedings or a few liquids. Steak and a baked potato; well, really, chicken, green beans and mashed potatoes, but still a major hurdle overcome on the long road to recovery.

A thousand miles away, my mother was able to eat with a fork for the first time in more than a year since she suffered serious head trauma, and it was a reason to rejoice.

Every day, three or four times, more or less, we sit down or belly up or stroll through the park, consuming the food that keeps us going. We take it for granted, this ability to eat, but for the very sick and badly injured, eating a normal diet, consumed in the normal way, is often the final step of a long journey.

When a body becomes very sick and its defense mechanisms are turned on to the max, the intestines, at that moment non-essential organs, are shut off; the body utilizes all its reserves to stay alive. Keep the heart pumping, send blood to the brain, but, those bowels, they'll be OK, at least for a short while. A failing heart, severe infection, or a bleeding body will usually have an associated paralytic ileus, a fancy word that means the bowels have been turned off, their presence unnecessary at that moment. That explains why people suffering heart attacks have nausea, or the badly injured, even if there are only broken bones, might vomit. This phenomenon might be transient, lasting only a few moments, or might persist for weeks.

During such times, normal eating becomes impossible, and food languishes in the stomach until it is rejected by an act of vomiting; nutrition must be supplied by alternative routes. If there is no external source, the body starts to consume itself. Glycogen stored in the liver is consumed, fat stores are depleted, and muscle is metabolized; our reserves are mobilized to keep vital organs functioning. Modern medicine, however, provides alternatives to such consumption. The individual who cannot eat can be fed intravenously, receiving thousands of calories, fluids, and complete nutrition via Total Parenteral Nutrition (TPN). If the GI tract is functional, but the patient is unable to eat, enteral feedings can be provided via tubes that pass through the nose into the stomach or directly through the abdominal wall into the stomach or small intestine, a bit more natural and physiologic than TPN but still a far cry from normal eating.

Normal eating. We take it for granted; I'm hungry, what's in the fridge or pantry or down the street at Millie's Diner? It seems our lives are built around the act of eating. We plan our meals for the day or week. Almost every new relationship starts with a shared meal or drink, "let's do lunch," or, "I'll meet you for dinner." In the OR, the director spends most of his or her time ensuring that the staff has "lunch" even if it's 9:00 a.m. or 4:00 p.m.

Eating in all its shapes and forms is essential to our being, just as breathing and sleeping are important to an individual's survival, and sex is important to the survival of the species. I have to say that we spend far more time on food and eating than we do on sex, perhaps a reflection of the relative importance of each endeavor.

The mechanics of eating; the consumption and digestion of food and drink certainly cannot be considered attractive, despite attempts to make such activities appear more refined. Our food is placed before us, on plates, in bowls, poured into glasses and mugs, ready for intake. We take up a knife and fork, or spoon; we raise a glass to our lips and receive our fare into our mouth.

The steak is chewed, the pasta slurped, the beans crushed, and then it is all washed down with a fine red wine. Each bite is savored by thousands of sensory receptors in our tongue, combined with our olfactory cells to convey taste to our brain; the tongue also provides the sense of texture and temperature, providing the complete package of gustatory splendor; the pleasure of eating.

Each organ that participates in this orgy of sensation plays a vital role. Starting with the eyes and the nose, we look for a pleasing appearance and aroma; both prepare the consumer for the pleasures of the repast that is forthcoming. Our lips, incredibly sensitive organs that are essential to eating and for demonstrating affection, receive the first sensation of temperature and texture as the food passes into the mouth, where the tongue mingles the sensations it receives with the aroma already received to convey the complete sense of taste to our brain. Powerful jaws and teeth tear and crush, mix and masticate, turning the once palatable dinner into a paste of appropriate consistency to be propelled to the oropharynx. Parotid, submandibular and numerous minor glands add saliva to soften and dilute the conglomeration, easing its passage from the oropharynx to the hypopharynx and finally propelled, by the coordinated action of several pharyngeal muscles, into the esophagus where the ingested mass begins its long journey through our body.

The stomach churns and mixes and further dilutes before delivering our once irresistible meal to the intestines for more complete digestion, leading to eventual absorption or expulsion. Our meal of steak, pasta, beans, and wine is transformed into fat on our hips, muscle on our arms, sugar in our liver, along with a number of other essential elements for our body, or passes out of our body, where it returns to the earth and might eventually be consumed again and the journey repeated

Such a complex process, repeated over and over and over. It's amazing that we never tire of eating, although we often seek variety: Italian, or Greek, or French, but even if we're stuffed to the gills, we manage to find room for that seven-layer chocolate cake. Eating might be our greatest pleasure; the act frequently performed in the public eye, shared with any and all.

Therefore, it's time to stand and applaud Lorraine's return from death's door to the realm of the healthy and whole. Every ingredient that is necessary for a body to eat and digest has resumed proper function, and soon she will be home with family and friends, enjoying a dinner at home or out. Although at this moment she might not appreciate it, the ability to eat is a great gift, one that should be cherished.

16. At Night

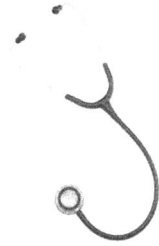

"The best cure for insomnia is to get a lot of sleep."
~ W. C. Fields

"I only need the pain med at night"; "I just take one a day, at night when I'm trying to sleep"; "I need something to help me at night"; I hear words like these over and over from patients. Something happens at night, lying in the dark, waiting for the escape of sleep to overtake us. The pain of recent surgery often intrudes and seems more intense at these moments. The distractions of the daytime, other people, the humdrum light and noise are gone, and all the pain that has been buried during waking hours rises to the surface.

Our brain is amazing, the way it filters out wave after wave of unwanted stimuli, selecting only what's important to capture our attention. But all this stimulation fades away in the night and we are left with only ourselves, our thoughts, dreams, and pains. My patients fill out a history questionnaire as part of their initial evaluation; one of the symptoms they can check is difficulty sleeping. I think almost half my patients check this box.

Little children cry out in fear, and their parents rush to comfort them; the darkness and solitude are fertile ground for the young imagination, calling up horrible monsters that prey on the innocent, but are frightened away by even the tiniest bit of light and a few sharp words from a loving parent.

The monsters of childhood give way to the demons of our later years. The worries of these supposedly enlightened and progressive times creep out during the dark hours, robbing us of the tranquility that sleep promises. Perhaps the monsters are real; a prodigal child, a wayward spouse, financial burdens, or disappointment over perceived failure, concerns that well up into our consciousness at a time when we yearn for the serenity and peace of sleep.

Charlie Brown of "Peanuts" fame would lie awake at night and ask questions out loud addressed to no one in particular or, perhaps, to God. The answers were never particularly comforting:

"Sometimes I lie awake at night and ask 'where did I go wrong?' And a voice answers 'This is going to take more than one night." - Charlie Brown in *Peanuts*

"Sometimes I lie awake at night and ask 'Why me?' And a voice answers, 'Nothing personal, your number just came up' - Charlie Brown in *Peanuts*

Is God so arbitrary? I doubt it.

But, the night isn't always bad. Triumphs and successes of the day bring a sense of joy and excitement that can keep us from the peace of sleep. It is far more likely that elation leads to celebration and sleep is banished for a while; our day-to-day struggles are pushed back into the recesses of our brain, quietly waiting for the moment to emerge and send our joyful feelings crashing into the abyss.

The Bible speaks of rest as a reward, something given by God for work well done.

"Come to Me, all you who labor and are heavy laden, and I will give you rest. Take My yoke upon you and learn from Me, for I am gentle and lowly in heart, and you will find rest for your souls. For My yoke is easy and My burden is light." - Matthew 11:28-30

At the end of a long day or a long life, God rewards us with His rest. Scripture presents rest as the ultimate gift from God. Over a six-day period God created the universe and our world, and on the seventh day, He rested. Number four of the Ten Commandments is to remember the Sabbath day and keep it holy, which means set apart as something special, a time for rest.

So night is the time for rest, to be alone with God and with our thoughts, a time of reflection on the day's events, and a time to anticipate the days to come. So many times at night I think about the day that has just passed, surgeries that have been done, family concerns, and any troubles. It's a time to offer prayers of thanks and supplication. Personally, I think God listens best at such moments, or, more likely, I can focus better at these times; the quiet darkness shields my thoughts from unwanted intrusion.

And then there's sleep. We drift away from consciousness, but remain alive. While we sleep, amazing things happen. Although it has never been proven, I think that sleep provides a time for repair: physical, mental, and emotional. Body temperature falls, heart rate decreases, blood pressure decreases, and vascular resistance falls. Our organs are bathed in blood that seems to circulate more slowly during sleep, allowing built-up toxins to be released from our cells and eliminated, focusing our immune system on potential invaders, repairing damages done, and probably a multitude of other functions that remain a mystery.

Sleep is the time for dreams, our pent-up thoughts and feelings released into a private theater that might be cryptic, vivid, heart-warming, or terrifying. Sometimes our dreams are in color, sometimes in black and white. Freud wrote a whole book on the interpretation of dreams. The Bible gave special credence to those who could interpret dreams and treated our dreams as messages from God. Daniel and Joseph were the premier dream interpreters of the Bible; they both suffered because of this skill, but they were also rewarded. Most often our dreams leave us confused, and often we forget them as soon as we awaken, leaving us with a vague recollection that something of importance might have transpired, but little more.

We might never remember a dream or remain oblivious to our environment, but we still yearn for sleep, for this time of physical, mental, emotional, and spiritual repair. We cannot live without its benefits, and yet it can prove to be so elusive. We lay awake, tossing and turning, counting sheep by the millions, downing pills and elixirs, searching for the elusive rest. Our world has become so complicated that moments to relax, do nothing, and dream become fleeting until they seem lost forever.

Where can we find peace? As children, the comforting word or touch of a parent was all that was needed. So, we come back to our Parent, to God, our Heavenly Father. His word, His grace, His promise are all that we need to find rest. It is promised throughout the Bible, and night is the time when we can feel His soothing touch and receive His peace.

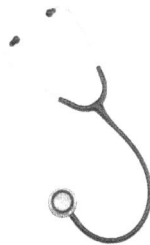

17. Walking the Halls

"What saves a man is to take a step. Then another step."

~ C. S. Lewis

I was walking down the hallway at one of the local hospitals today and a patient was wheeled by in her bed, attended by a nurse, respiratory therapist, and patient aide. The patient lay to one side, a tube exiting her nose, the end clamped and sitting next to her head; she was still, and her cheeks were noticeably sunken. She didn't appear to be extremely elderly, perhaps in her 60s, but she had the vacant stare of someone waiting for the inevitability of death. Her look contrasted sharply with those attending to her needs. Idle chatter between the nurse, therapist, and aide suggested they were oblivious to the patient in their charge.

But, in a moment it all changed. An irregular "beep...beep" sang out from the monitor, and they all turned to the patient. The respiratory therapist checked the oxygen while the nurse addressed the patient, "Mrs. X, can you hear me...are you OK?" A weak smile emanated from Mrs. X, who nodded her head as if to say, "Yes, I'm alright." All the while, the patient aide felt Mrs. X's pulse. Satisfied that Mrs. X was not in any danger, the team continued on their way to their destination.

I was struck by this brief exchange between patient and caregivers. It is far too easy for doctors and patients to overlook the amazing professionalism that is found among hospital staff. The army of nurses, patient aides, respiratory therapists, physical therapists, occupational therapists, speech pathologists, EKG technicians, phlebotomists, lab technicians, surgical technicians and any other ancillary help that I might have omitted, keeps the hospital running smoothly and, more than anything, helps our patients return to good health.

The scenes in the hallway vary from moment to moment, but most have one thing in common; everyone involved is doing their utmost to help a sick or injured individual return to a normal life. It is amazing that patients with tubes coming out of every available body orifice, receiving IV infusions of medicine designed to keep their failing heart pumping, or on ventilators, are whisked from place to place at all hours of the day or night, without mishap. Sometimes the situation is dire. Unstable trauma patients often need transport from ER to OR, or to the ICU. There might be an ER nurse or technician holding direct pressure on a bleeding artery, while others pump in blood, monitor vital signs, ventilate, or merely drive. Maneuvering a large bed or stretcher laden with pumps and IV's hanging on wobbly poles, while administering to a patient's needs and keeping an eye on the whole situation, is a remarkable feat, and, more amazingly, one that has become routine.

As I cruised down the hallways, I encountered a variety of individuals. Patients dressed in robes and hospital attire, urinary catheters clipped to the gown, IV pole in tow, walking from here to there, nowhere in particular, doing their best to follow doctor's orders to "get up and walk." Then there are the physical therapists, walking along side patients, the commonly seen strap around the patient's waist, sometimes with walkers or the occasional crutches, starting their patients on the road to normal locomotion.

The simple act of walking. It is one of the things that separates humanity from all other animals. There are other animals that stand upright, such as kangaroos, birds, and some rats, but none of them travel for any significant distance by walking. Kangaroos and similar beasts hop from place to place; birds can walk, but primarily fly; the great apes are able to walk upright, but use their arms far more than their legs. Bipedal walking, placing one foot in front of the other, is the sole province of mankind. I can't say that this makes *Homo Sapiens* superior, but it does set us apart.

The mechanism is straightforward. The brain and spinal cord send signals to the muscles of the lower extremity, and locomotion is initiated. Sensory nerves provide information on distance, slope, and friction levels of the surface, and appropriate pressure and strength is applied to propel the individual forward, backward, or sideways. Sensory and motor systems also work together to maintain balance. Change the muscles utilized and increase the force generated, and running occurs. The fastest human runners can reach speeds of about 24 mph, far short of the speeds reached by the fastest land animal, the cheetah, at 70 mph, or the fastest birds, reaching top speeds of 170 mph.

Locomotion is important to the surgical patient. Orthopedic surgeons want their hip replacement or fracture patients up and walking as soon as possible. Those of us in General Surgery are always admonishing our patients to get up and walk. We believe that it helps restore normal GI tract function more quickly, while lowering the incidence of respiratory complications. Venous blood flow is augmented by the pumping action provided by muscular contraction; the contraction squeezing the veins, propelling the blood, while the venous valves keep the flow towards the heart. Immobility leads to venous stasis and increases the incidence of venous thrombosis, a common post-surgical complication.

And, it is natural for humans to be ambulatory. I suppose that in prehistoric days, when predators were common, humans who lost their locomotive skills became easy prey. Nowadays, those of us who lose the ability to walk become prey to a different sort of predator: venous thrombosis, pneumonia, de-conditioning, bed sores, and other maladies, all consequences of immobility.

In my surgical practice, the ability to get up and walk is one of the criteria utilized to decide if a patient is ready to leave the hospital. When a patient is able to get up and walk, has normal vital signs (pulse, blood pressure, respirations, and temperature), is able to eat, and has normal bowel and urinary function, it usually means he or she is well enough to be home. It is not surprising that many chronically ill patients find it difficult to reach such a goal. Walking is often the most difficult to achieve. But, walking allows us to be independent, and for many of our patients, independence is a thing to be cherished and maintained, often above everything else.

18. Looking Cool

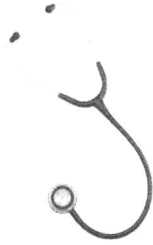

"A lot of people are obsessed with looking cool. They feel they have to look after their image."
~ Adrian Edmondson

When I was in medical school, during my surgical clerkship, I was introduced to a large number of surgeons from a variety of different specialties. I always found the actual surgery to be fascinating, which is one reason I decided to specialize in this area. But, I also was fascinated by the surgeons. They all seemed so confident and comfortable in the OR, as if they were born to be there. In those early years, I also noticed that there were certain things that the surgeons did that looked "cool." I distinctly remember being impressed by one surgeon's ability to orient a needle exactly how he wanted it by manipulating it with only the needle holder. To my neophyte eyes, this was the ultimate cool; recently I started thinking, again, about what it takes to look "cool" in the OR.

The cool OR façade begins with appearance; properly styled, slightly form-fitting scrubs, preferably monogrammed or inscribed with the individual's logo, are a must. Designer scrubs are most cool for women. Scrubs that are too tight or too loose are a no-no. Scrub bottoms that are pulled too high or hang too low are definitely uncool. Even slightly different color variation between tops and bottoms disqualify the wearer from membership in the cool surgeon fraternity. Men should sport surgical caps jauntily worn slightly to the side. Bouffant style head covering is not acceptable for male surgeons, which leaves me among the uncool. Women may wear the bouffant style, but custom designed ones are required. There are no requisite shoes to be amongst the cool, although clogs tend towards being cool.

The real test of coolness comes during the operation. The aforementioned ability to manipulate a needle without holding it is still way cool. Holding multiple instruments on one hand is also considered essential cool. This skill involves putting your ring finger through ringed handle of scissors and/or clamps and flipping them back out of the way while operating with a different instrument. One instrument on the ring ringer qualifies for mild coolness, two brings the surgeon to the intermediate level, three raises him or her to expert, and four means membership in the exclusive "superstar" club. Of course, any fumbling at any time, no matter how many instruments are involved, demotes the surgeon to completely uncool status. Similarly, attempting to manipulate the needle sans hands, being unsuccessful, and then having to use fingers to adjust it also is very uncool. As a resident, one particular attending physician repeatedly tried to teach me to hold instruments on my ring finger instead of putting them down, which was my preference. He wasn't really trying to teach me to be cool; he was trying to teach me to be efficient and avoid wasted motion. I never really mastered this skill; I still put the instruments down when I'm not using them and exchange them as necessary. I guess I'm still making unnecessary wasted movements. I don't think my patients have suffered because of this deficiency.

Music played in the OR also can be a major contributor to achieving the proper state of coolness. Heavy Metal Rock 'n Roll played at over 100 decibels is supposed to be cool, while country western is not far behind. Listening to Swiss yodeling, classical music (my preference), or no music is not cool and also relegates me to the uncool category.

Being cool in the OR has the potential for all sorts of benefits. Having one's choice of surgical techs and nurses is one perk. Being forgiven rude or ill-tempered behavior also seems to be the province of the "cool" surgeon. Charming the OR scheduler to get a favorable start time for surgery also comes much easier to the coolest surgeons.

After thinking about all this coolness, I realize that nothing I do fits into the aforementioned cool category. But, there are some things that surgeons do that are *really, really, really* cool: treating the surgical staff with the greatest respect, being attentive to the worries and needs of the patient before, during, and after surgery, and making their families fully aware of what has or might transpire throughout the course of surgery. All these are the true epitome of coolness.

Throwing instruments, belittling and berating staff, and ignoring patients and their families' questions and concerns, are definitely uncool. The coolest surgeons put patients first, do what's right whether it's the middle of the day or 2:00 a.m. Doing the right operation, at the right time, and staying on top of any bumps in the surgical journey is what's truly cool. All the rest is empty window dressing.

However, being able to flip the needle around with just the needle holder still looks pretty cool.

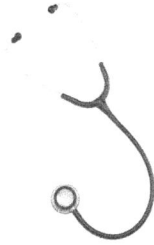

19. Surgical Deficiency

"He who is proficient in learning, but deficient in morals, is more deficient than proficient."

~ Unknown

It has recently been brought to my attention that certain skills that many surgeons consider absolutely vital to success are lacking from my repertoire. Elective courses in medical school and residency equipped many surgeons with certain knowledge and abilities that I am completely lacking. My sense of fair play and the need for complete disclosure mandate that I make this report. Listed here are those courses I failed to take during my surgical training, vital lessons that might make me wholly inadequate to practice surgery.

Instrument Throwing 101 and 102
A two-semester course that instructs the surgical resident in the proper technique for throwing an instrument off the operative field. The first semester

covers blunt instruments, such as clamps and forceps, while the second part instructs on the proper technique for hurling sharp instruments, scalpels, needles, and scissors. Proficiency in the short Mayo toss, the medium range Anesthesia throw, and the long range Nurse hurl is expected by the completion. Final exam is judged on accuracy of the throw, amount of disorder created, and physical and emotional damage inflicted. Measurement of stress is also graded.

Tantrums 100

A one-semester course offered as part of the medical school curriculum, tantrums will provide the student an introduction to those situations where an outburst is considered appropriate and necessary, differing tantrum techniques, and proper targets. An extensive video collection, demonstrating everything from the red-faced huff to the hot air tempest, is required viewing. Final exam will be part oral, grading quantity and quality of the student's angry fit, and part practical, measuring the negative impact on a recipient subject: nurse, technician, patient, family member, or hospital administrator.

Condescension 330

This is an upper level course which has Tantrums 100 as a prerequisite. Advanced techniques of sarcasm, insulting, and belittling are taught. Extra credit work in racial, gender, and sexual preference slurring is available. Final exam is written: true or false, and multiple choice.

Physical Assault 600

A graduate level course open only to those who have successfully completed all the above courses. Appropriate technique for pushing, bruising, and surreptitious sexual harassment are taught by experts in each area. The first half of the course is didactic classroom work, while the second half includes field training in the OR, ICU, and patient ward. Passing this course will be at the discretion of the instructing faculty, but any arrests, indictments, or lawsuits will be grounds for summary failure.

Far too often stories of such inappropriate behavior surface. Any such behavior detracts from patient care and leads to an atmosphere of tension in the OR and other patient care areas. Everyone who works in the healthcare arena has a shared goal of taking the best possible care of the sick and injured patients who come under our care. There is no place for inappropriate actions and behavior. I apologize for my lack of skill in these areas.

20. Medical Terms

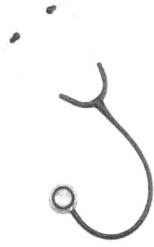

"Words are only postage stamps delivering the object for you to unwrap."

~ George Bernard Shaw

Antiseptic: the woman married to Uncle Septic

X-Ray: pornographic picture

Cine X-Ray: pornographic movie

CAT Scan: Imaging a patient by running a feline over their body

PET Scan: Similar to CAT Scan, except a variety of animals may be used

Perirectal: in and around a lizard or snake

Clamp: a pain in your side that develops while exercising

Ultrasound: a noise that can only be heard by dogs

Operation: A children's game that asks the contestant to remove the "wishbone," "spare ribs," etc.

ICU: looking at someone

Surgeon: a large fresh-water fish

Tumor: one less than three more

Carcinoma: Short for leaving one's automobile in Omaha

Cervical: a British nobleman named "Vic" for short

Thyroid: a hemorrhoid on the upper leg

Appendix: a program for iPhone

Kidney: part of a child's leg

Rectum: stopping short of killin' em

Resect: have intercourse again

Anal: to dissolve a marriage

Duct: feathered, web-footed water fowl

Spinal Cord: a collection of musical notes

Lung: reaching for an object

Lymphatic: physically dependent on tree branches

Hypoglossal: not very shiny

Vagus: not very definite

Peritoneal: Two Irish brothers

Gastric: a joke performed with flatus

Parathyroid: two hemorrhoids on an upper leg

Bile Duct: to purchase a feathered, web-footed water fowl

Bunion: an onion roll

Metacarpal: to encounter a scavenging fish while swimming

Humerus: funny

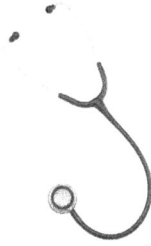

21. Triumph

"Triumphs without difficulties are empty. Indeed; it is difficulties that make the triumph. It is no feat to travel the smooth road."

~ Unknown

Over the years I've had some patients who arrived at the hospital very sick, almost dead, but managed to walk out of the hospital completely whole and on the road to 100% recovery. Sometimes this would require a quick trip to surgery, and sometimes it was the decision not to operate that allowed them to carry on.

Don't operate. A surprising statement, coming from a surgeon. After all, the old saying has always been, "To cut is to cure." But sometimes, it is prudent to wait and see.

Rhonda came to the hospital complaining of severe abdominal pain, one episode of bloody diarrhea and bloating. She had a past medical history significant for two previous myocardial infarctions (heart attacks), congestive heart failure, peripheral vascular disease with two previous lower extremity bypass surgeries, and hemolytic anemia, which was currently being treated with steroids. She had been in the hospital for about eighteen hours when I was called. During those eighteen hours, she had received only nominal IV fluid resuscitation, IV antibiotics, and had been kept NPO (nothing by mouth).

She had a metabolic acidosis and her abdomen was diffusely tender when I examined her. Abdominal and pelvic CT scan revealed dilated bowel, primarily the large bowel, which did not appear inflamed or thickened. There was report of air in the biliary tree, presumably from a previous biliary tract procedure, the history of which could be neither confirmed nor denied. She was awake and alert, her pulmonary status was normal, and her renal function was normal.

With her history of severe vascular disease, acidosis, bloody diarrhea, and the physical findings, my diagnosis was ischemic colitis. I was asked by the ICU nurse, "When are you going to operate?" I answered hopefully never. Poor Rhonda was extremely high risk for a variety of severe, life-threatening complications with any major surgical procedure. At the same time, she had the very real possibility that her bowel was already gangrenous rather than merely potentially reversible ischemia. She had not had adequate fluid resuscitation at that point. No matter what was ultimately done, such therapy had to come first. If she continued to have a metabolic acidosis, if her abdomen remained tender, if other signs of severe sepsis persisted, then there was no question surgery would be needed to save her life.

However, I waited and watched, very, very closely. Her white blood cell count, which had been very high at 32,000 on admission and had decreased to 24,000 by the time I was called, continued to decrease, to 19,000. This could be a good sign or a bad sign. Good if it meant that her sepsis was responding favorably to the therapeutic intervention, bad if it meant that her white blood cells were being consumed by overwhelming severe infection. A follow up plain abdominal X-Ray revealed pneumatosis intestinale, which is air in the wall of the bowel, a sign of ischemia, but something that is reversible if the ischemic process is reversed.

Wait a bit longer; her acidosis resolved, her renal function remained normal, she had a normal bowel movement, her tenderness diminished, all over the first 36 hours. She then developed respiratory distress requiring endotracheal intubation and ventilator support, but this also resolved. She also occluded her previous bilateral femoral popliteal bypass grafts, but her feet remained adequately perfused.

Follow-up testing revealed that the changes in the colon resolved. The initial finding of air in the biliary tree was reinterpreted as air in the portal venous system, a condition only seen when there is some sort of severe intraabdominal catastrophe, but this also had completely resolved.

Her pulmonary status gradually improved and she was weaned from the ventilator, was able to start eating, and was moved from the ICU to a regular room. Although she had arterial occlusions in her legs, her collateral circulation was adequate to maintain the viability of her feet. As she recovered and was transferred to the Rehab unit, she did have some pain in her legs when she walked, probably due to the arterial occlusive disease in her legs, a condition that would be addressed at a later time, after she had recovered from her septic event.

Looking back at this case, major therapeutic decisions were required at almost every moment. What was the diagnosis? How should she be treated? Does she need additional steroids? And the biggest question: Should she undergo surgery?

I was convinced that her chance of surviving a major surgery, given her overall condition was poor. However, if it seemed that she had developed an intraabdominal event that was irreversible and immediately life-threatening, surgical intervention would have been the only option. In Rhonda's case, she never quite reached this level. I was firmly convinced that the diagnosis was ischemic colitis. The underlying pathophysiology of this condition is usually a combination of poor GI tract perfusion, often related to heart failure or dehydration, coupled with underlying vascular disease. Of course, a sudden occlusion of a major intestinal mesenteric vessel can cause this condition or cause frank gangrene. The GI tract, however, has excellent collateral circulation such that even complete occlusion of one or even two of the major arteries, Celiac, Superior Mesenteric, or Inferior Mesenteric artery, might be well tolerated with the development of no, or minimal, symptoms. In this case, it is likely that Rhonda occluded one of these vessels and developed ischemic changes in her colon. This is what precipitated her illness. However, once appropriate treatment was instituted and collateral flow improved, these ischemic changes resolved. Although she did develop some immediate complications of the initial ischemic event, she ultimately recovered, although not without sequelae that would require intervention at a later date.

A similar case, but one managed in a different way was Shirley. Shirley was a 60-year-old lady who came to the ER complaining of abdominal pain for nine days. She had a history of chronic back pain and regularly took high doses of narcotic pain medication to control her pain; she also had a history of Chronic Obstructive Pulmonary Disease (COPD, emphysema related to cigarette smoking). I was called by the ER physician shortly after her arrival. The history he reported was that she'd had pain for nine days, had eaten almost nothing during that time, and had been taking her pain medication for the abdominal pain. Her abdomen was very tender, and the ER doctor was sure she was going to need surgery. The obligatory CT scan had not been done yet; she was to go shortly.

When he called, I was about to start a surgery at another hospital; therefore, I asked him to call me back after the CT scan was done, and I would come to see her then. The CT scan was reported as unremarkable with no acute findings. I saw her a short time later; she was in the ICU, sitting up, reporting that her pain seemed to be diminished. She was receiving appropriate fluid resuscitation and overall seemed to be much improved over her initial presentation. She gave a very vague history of abdominal pain with associated nausea which, as previously reported, had started nine days before admission. Her exam revealed mild diffuse abdominal tenderness and signs of dehydration. I reviewed the CT scan with the Radiologist; neither one of us saw anything that suggested an intraabdominal catastrophe. Watchful waiting began. She seemed to improve considerably that first day. Her initial tachycardia (rapid heart rate) improved, her pain decreased, but she still had periods of hypotension (low blood pressure), suggesting there was an ongoing problem.

Her abdominal exam remained equivocal, had no definite signs of peritonitis, but still revealed some tenderness. She also developed respiratory compromise and required endotracheal intubation and ventilator support. I was still concerned about a possible intraabdominal source, and I repeated her abdominal CT scan. Once again, nothing significantly abnormal was reported, although when I reviewed the films with the Radiologist, we both thought the colon might have become somewhat thickened, a sign of inflammation. Her WBC count was rising, going from 17,000 to 28,000. Her abdominal exam seemed a little more tender, and she was more hypotensive. At this point, I made the decision that surgery was necessary. It was becoming apparent that she was developing worsening sepsis, and survival would be unlikely without some sort of intervention.

The surgery that was performed was a total abdominal colectomy with creation of an ileostomy. The colon appeared inflamed, but not obviously gangrenous. Everything else in her abdomen appeared healthy. She improved considerably after this surgery.

Her blood pressure stabilized, and her WBC count came down from 28,000 to 15,000, and then to 10,000. Her pulmonary status gradually improved, and she was able to leave the hospital about three weeks later. Subsequently, I operated on her and reversed her ileostomy, reconnecting the small intestine to her rectum. She now has to live with having four to five bowel movements a day, a consequence of having almost no colon, but otherwise she is well.

Shirley was a case of vigilance, paying close attention to all the various parameters that are monitored in very ill patients, and intervening when conditions change. One could argue that surgery should have been done when she arrived, and, in retrospect that might be true. But, it's also true that an early operation might have missed the pathology, that the severe colitis that developed might not have been apparent early in her hospitalization. This could have led to an inadequate colon resection. What is very apparent is that when Shirley started to go downhill, there was no choice but to operate. Any more watchful waiting would have allowed her to reach a point of inevitable death, something physicians try to avoid if at all possible.

Some surgical conditions that are encountered require paying close attention to details that may seem trivial, but which sometimes spell the difference between life and death.

Connie presented with complaints of abdominal pain, nausea, and vomiting for three days. She initially had some diarrhea, but then stopped passing anything, neither stool nor flatus. She had undergone a hysterectomy twenty years before this admission. Her CT scan revealed typical findings of Small Bowel Obstruction, and the clinical picture supported this diagnosis. I was called to see her the morning after her admission. She stated that her pain was diminished, but she still had intermittent cramps. Her abdominal exam revealed only mild tenderness, which was not localized to any one area. She was a bit tachycardic; her heart rate was 110. Her WBC count on admission was mildly elevated at 12,800, and a repeat had not been done. Review of her CT scan confirmed that the appearance was of a small bowel obstruction.

There are always questions that arise when evaluating a patient with intestinal obstruction: Is this a partial obstruction, which would be more likely to resolve without surgery; or a high grade or complete obstruction, which almost certainly would require surgical intervention? Are there signs of bowel ischemia: Tachycardia, usually a heart rate over 120; significantly elevated WBC count, greater than 18,000; localized tenderness or mass suggestive of gangrenous bowel; or persistent metabolic acidosis? Other questions that might be asked are: Has the patient had previous surgery? Is the obstruction in the small bowel or large bowel? The large bowel, having a much greater resident population of bacteria, presents a greater urgency when it is completely obstructed.

In the case of Connie, she didn't really have signs of intestinal ischemia. She did, however, appear to have a high-grade obstruction and she was tachycardic, a bit more than I would have expected with an uncomplicated small bowel obstruction. The decision was made to operate. I informed her admitting physician. He asked me if I planned to operate that day, which was Friday, or wait until Monday. Once the decision is made that a patient with intestinal obstruction requires surgery it is most prudent to proceed with surgery expeditiously, and Connie was taken to surgery that day. In Connie's case her prompt surgery was most fortunate.

Upon opening her abdomen, bloody fluid was encountered immediately, never a good sign. She had the expected dilated small bowel which was followed down into her pelvis where the expected adhesive bands tethering the bowel were discovered. These were snipped and the bowel was freed from the pelvis. At this point I found what I had been expecting from the moment I encountered the bloody fluid in her abdomen. The terminal ileum, which is the last part of the small bowel before it continues on into the colon, was gangrenous (dead). It had been adherent in the pelvis and had twisted around the adhesion, what is termed a volvulus. This gangrenous bowel was resected and the small bowel anastamosed to the right colon. She had an uneventful post-operative course and made a complete recovery.

In this case there were few signs to suggest she had such a severe, life-threatening condition. The only true sign was her tachycardia, something that was present since the time of her arrival to the hospital. The fact that she was feeling less pain was misleading, and only persistent questioning revealed that she still had symptoms of high-grade obstruction. The fact that it was Friday and I would be off for the weekend also might have contributed to my decision to operate; I'm really not sure. Sometimes it's best to be lucky.

Another case that could be called a triumph is Manfred. He was 85 years old, still going to work as an inspector at one of the local chemical plants, had a history of Congestive Heart Failure and cardiac arrhythmias, with a permanent pacemaker. I was called to see him because he was hypoxic and his chest X-Ray and CT scan revealed that his stomach or colon had herniated into his left chest. The initial report from the ER physician, at about midnight, was that he was stable, receiving supplemental oxygen, and that his evaluation could wait until morning. Trusting this evaluation, I saw Manfred at about 8:00 a.m. What I found was an elderly man struggling with every breath, with completely absent breath sounds on the left side. It was true that his stomach had herniated into his left chest, and it was nearly completely compressing his left lung. A chest X-Ray from six months prior revealed no such hernia. Poor Manfred was working on only one lung; this in a man who already had pretty significant underlying cardiac disease with very minimal reserve function.

There was no question that he needed immediate surgery. Despite some misgivings from the Anesthesiologist, Manfred underwent emergency surgery to return his stomach to its rightful position in the abdomen and repair the hiatal hernia. It was like night and day once the massively dilated stomach was delivered from the chest into the abdomen. All of a sudden, his oxygen saturation shot up to 100% from

92, ventilation became much easier, his blood pressure stabilized, his heart rate diminished from 110 to 76. The herniated stomach had dilated to about four times normal size. In retrospect it is likely that over a period of days, air had become trapped in his stomach which at some point over the previous six months had herniated through the esophageal hiatus, creating what is called a paraesophageal hiatal hernia.

This condition can be contrasted with the far more common sliding hiatal hernia. Sliding hernias move up and down through the esophageal hiatus; they are often associated with gastroesophageal reflux, but rarely lead to complications such as Manfred's, which was an incarcerated stomach, or to gastric volvulus, which is twisting of the stomach. The paraesophageal type of hernia is characterized by the gastroesophageal junction being in its normal position below the diaphragm, while the stomach or other abdominal viscera herniates through the hiatus, alongside the normally positioned GE junction.

As Manfred's stomach continued to inflate, like a balloon, his left lung became compressed until a critical point was reached, he could barely breathe, and he finally felt the need to seek medical attention. If he had further delayed going to the doctor, or if surgery had been delayed, the stomach could have perforated, which probably would have been fatal. As it turned out, he recovered uneventfully and left the hospital after about one week.

Over the years, such triumphs of medicine over disease have been common. Sometimes luck plays a role, far more often careful watchfulness and attention to details are most important. Sometimes a patient's recovery is completely unexpected, a defiance of the odds; such patients get to live and fight another day. And, sometimes, everything is done exactly right, by the book, but the patient still dies. Such are the vicissitudes of the fine art of medicine and surgery.

22. Disaster

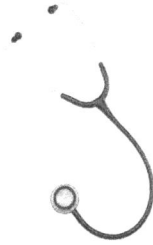

"If I could learn to treat triumph and disaster the same, then I would find bliss."

~ Kathie Lee Gifford

I've written over and over that the practice of surgery requires constant attention to detail, vigilance, and decision-making such that surgeons step in and do their job at the appropriate time and in the proper manner. The vast majority of the time, the outcome is extremely favorable, with complete recovery and excellent long-term results. However, sometimes the best intentions lead to disaster. Over the years, some patients stand out as particularly tragic.

Harold was a 28-year-old man who had suffered a fractured femur in a skiing accident. Unfortunately, his initial treatment had failed, and he was left with a nonunion of his fracture. He was referred to the Plastic Surgery service at the hospital I was at during my fourth year of residency. The Chief Resident on the Plastic Surgery service scheduled him for a procedure called a free fibula flap. The intent of this operation was to replace what was likely devascularized bone that wouldn't heal with new, healthy bone that had its own blood supply. The Plastic surgeons would harvest the fibula with its vascular pedicle, remove the bad bone, replace it with the new bone, and connect those normal blood vessels to those in the area. This new, healthy bone would then heal the fracture and Harold would be able to return to his normal, everyday, ambulatory life.

The big day of surgery came and Harold went under anesthesia at 7:30 a.m. The surgery went on and on and on. I was curious about what was taking so long, but I wasn't involved at this point, except as an interested bystander. Harold finally emerged from the OR at 7:30 a.m. the following morning. I made some not so discreet inquiries as to the reasons the surgery had taken such a long time.

It turns out that the initial part of the operation had proceeded without a hitch, that is, preparing the site of the nonunion to accept the flap and harvesting of the fibula and its associated blood supply. However, when the fibula was sewn into place and the arterial and venous anastomoses performed, the bone was put in upside down, which led to the artery being anastamosed to the vein and the vein being anastamosed to the artery. This obviously didn't work and it had to be redone. Apparently, after it was reoriented and sewn into place, it still wasn't right. The perfusion of the flap was poor and attempts to redo it were unsuccessful. Finally, the fibula was left in place as a free graft and the surgery was terminated. But, Harold's problems were only beginning.

Once settled in the ICU, Harold immediately manifested signs of respiratory failure. He became difficult to oxygenate, and his airway pressures became very high, signs of Adult Respiratory Distress Syndrome. The Plastic Surgery service consulted our General Surgery service for ICU care, and, before the day was out, Harold came under the care of the General Surgery consultants, myself and my two co-consultants, we being the three fourth-year residents responsible for consultations. Poor Harold only became sicker and sicker. It became increasingly difficult to ventilate him. He required extremely high levels of PEEP, which stands for Positive End Expiratory Pressure. PEEP increases the pressure in airways, which improves oxygenation, but at the price of decreasing blood flow through the lungs and to the rest of the body.

Harold's airway pressures reached 120, which is extremely high; normal airway pressures are around 20 or so. He repeatedly set off the alarms because his pressures exceeded the scale on the ventilators. His leg surgery failed miserably and became infected; he developed ischemia of his operated leg and evaluation revealed that he had thrombosed the Superficial Femoral Artery in the operated leg. Review of his pre-operative arteriogram revealed a 50-60% stenosis in this artery, narrowing that the Plastic Surgeons had not considered significant. At this point, it became very significant. In the face of an infected wound and a patient barely alive, the only alternative for what had become frank gangrene of his right leg was amputation above the knee. After this was done, he was officially transferred to the Vascular Surgery service. He remained very sick, but was holding on. His lungs slowly improved. He did require a tracheostomy, but eventually he recovered enough to be weaned from the ventilator, begin eating, and initiate physical therapy.

However, attempts to remove his tracheostomy were met with repeated failure. He would become short of breath and the tube would have to be reinserted. Evaluation of his upper airway demonstrated tracheal stenosis, a condition that would require another surgery.

He underwent this surgery about a month later and during that operation suffered injury to both of his recurrent laryngeal nerves. These two nerves innervate the muscles which move the vocal cords and, if injured, result in vocal cord paralysis. Poor Harold had to have his tracheostomy redone to provide an adequate airway. From start to finish, Harold suffered the worst of complications following what was a semi-elective surgery. He ended up absent his right leg, with a permanent tracheostomy, and possibly permanently diminished lung capacity. I never actually operated on him (luckily), although I was involved in his care at various points along the way.

Candace was an elderly woman, under the care of another surgeon, with abdominal pain caused by gallstones. This was in the early days of laparoscopic surgery, a time when many of the established surgeons were struggling to master this new technique. She underwent a laparoscopic cholecystectomy, which is gallbladder removal utilizing tiny incisions.

Immediately after surgery she complained of severe pain, but she'd just had surgery, so this was not completely unexpected. Her pain persisted for the next 48 hours. She was treated with appropriate analgesics, but then developed shortness of breath and hypotension. She was transferred to the ICU. Evaluation at that time suggested she might have had a pulmonary embolus (a blood clot that travels to the lungs), and she was started on heparin, a powerful blood thinner. However, she developed serious bleeding shortly after starting this medication and she was returned to surgery.

During the course of her evaluation, she did have an abdominal CT scan which suggested that there was leakage of GI fluids from the duodenum, which is the first part of the small intestine, into the peritoneal cavity. However, when she was returned to the OR, her surgeon did not notice the perforation of her duodenum. He did find massive bleeding from the liver bed, the area where the gallbladder had resided until her initial surgery. The surgeon decided to pack this area to tamponade the bleeding, appropriate management of such a complication, particularly for patients who are on blood thinners. He used Kerlex gauze for the packing. This type of gauze is frequently used for a variety of dressings, but it is usually not used intraoperatively because it lacks a radiopaque marker. Such markers make things visible on X-Rays. All of the sponges utilized during surgery have such markers; in case one is left inside of a patient it can be detected by X-Ray.

After her second operation Candace's family arrived, upset and angry. The patient had never informed them she was having surgery, and now she'd suffered severe complications. At this point, she was in the ICU, on a ventilator, requiring infusion of pressors (medication to elevate the blood pressure). In the evening on the day following her second operation, I received a call from one of the consultants on the case asking if I would see the patient. Her family had lost confidence in the original surgeon. I agreed and came to see her in the ICU and talk with her family.

She was just as described, on a ventilator, blood pressure around 100/40, heart rate 115, oxygen saturation in the mid 90's. Her right subcostal wound was packed with Kerlex gauze and there was small amount of serosanguinous drainage, fluid that would be expected to drain from an open abdominal wound. I told her family she was very ill and would need to be returned to the OR at some point to remove the packing. However, after reviewing all the records, I wasn't convinced that bleeding had been the primary problem.

I called her original surgeon, and he presented everything that had transpired. Specifically, he told me he had packed two Kerlex gauze rolls in the gallbladder bed to control bleeding and advised me to leave them in place for five days. I thanked him for his advice and then went to review the X-Rays and labs. Her hemoglobin level had actually gone up on the day after surgery, which would be very unusual in a patient with significant bleeding. The CT scan demonstrated contrast material mixed with the fluid that had collected in her gallbladder fossa, beneath the liver. Such a finding can be seen either with very brisk bleeding, which she'd had, or with contrast leaking from the GI tract. Her chart stated that she complained of severe pain and required increasingly higher doses of Demerol. Finally, when she became unstable, some intervention began.

I talked with her family and told them that I thought she needed to return to the OR sooner than five days. It was late at night, and I scheduled her for exploratory laparotomy for the following morning.

At surgery, I initially removed the Kerlex packs, making sure that two were removed. There was no active bleeding. However, I was surprised to find a large amount of bile in the abdomen. My thought at this point was that there was an injury to the Common Bile Duct, the main duct that connects the Liver to the intestine. However, I did not find any bile duct injury; what I did find was a hole in the duodenum, which explained the bilious fluid. I repaired and patched this and left a drain.

After this operation, Candace gradually improved. She did develop respiratory failure and was on the ventilator for about two weeks. She eventually was transferred to one of the Long Term Acute Care hospitals where I'd see her on a weekly basis. She never completely recovered and had difficulty eating. She was reevaluated with a CT scan of her abdomen and a new abscess was demonstrated.

This time I consulted with my friendly Interventional Radiologist who percutaneously drained the abscess, which was in front of her stomach, well away from the area of her previous surgery. Unfortunately, the abscess never completely resolved. As a matter of fact, the CT appearance changed very little after the drainage. She had persistent fever and nausea. It soon became obvious that she would need another surgery.

The following day she returned to the operating theater. I approached her through the midline, which was right over the site of the abscess. As soon as I entered the peritoneal cavity I discovered why the abscess never got any smaller. Sitting in the middle of this abscess, in front of the stomach and far away from the gallbladder fossa or the duodenum was a Kerlex roll. It was apparent that three rolls had been used to pack the abdomen when she was bleeding, not two. I don't know why only two had been reported and I don't know why this one had been placed well away from the area that had been bleeding. What I do know is that this final operation was too much for poor Candace. She did not tolerate this surgery very well, developed multi-organ failure, and eventually succumbed.

There were some lessons learned from poor Candace. The first is to pay attention to the patient. She complained of very severe pain after surgery; pain far greater than what is expected after a "routine" laparoscopic cholecystectomy, and the pain persisted. I frequently see patients complain of severe pain the first few hours after such an operation, but it almost always improves considerably after two to three hours. Candace's pain only worsened. The lesson learned is that pain out of proportion to what's expected demands some sort of evaluation. This could be simple blood tests or more in depth radiographic examination.

The second lesson is that surgeons should always look to the site of the operation for the cause of post-operative complications. Candace was treated for pulmonary embolus, which required giving her heparin to anticoagulate her. This almost surely precipitated the bleeding that occurred. All along, however, the problem was really a perforated duodenum. Such a condition explains the severe pain she suffered, and the rise in her hemoglobin level seen on the first post-operative day and most everything else that developed.

Third, if one is going to pack the abdomen to control bleeding, it is important to remember how many packs are used and to use material that has an appropriate radiopaque marker, so that it isn't left behind. Surgical Lap pads are best for this purpose.

Now, I don't want you to think that I've never had any disaster of my own making. Let me tell you about Jack.

Jack was 76 years old and came to see me after being diagnosed with cancer of the esophagus. He had been treated initially with Radiation therapy and chemotherapy and now was ready for surgery. His tumor was located in the lower third of the esophagus, about 3 cm above the gastroesophageal junction. The surgery that was planned was an esophageal resection which would involve abdominal and thoracic (chest) incisions. The stomach is mobilized so that it can be brought up into the chest to replace the cancerous segment of esophagus that is removed. The stomach, and its blood supply, can actually be mobilized so that it can easily reach to the level of the neck. I am not a thoracic surgeon; therefore, I enlisted the aid of my partner, who did do chest surgery.

The surgery was progressing uneventfully. I freed the stomach without difficulty; the thoracic portion was uncomplicated; the diseased segment of esophagus was not adherent to any surrounding structures; the Pathologist reported that the margins of the resection were free of cancer; and the esophageal-gastric anastomosis went well. All that was left was an expected uneventful recovery.

Unfortunately, that was not to be. Jack, initially, seemed to be recovering fairly well. There were a few minor respiratory issues, which were addressed, but nothing else that suggested he was in for anything but a smooth post-operative course.

The first setback came on the third day after surgery when the pathology report was completed. Pathological examination had revealed that there was tumor present at the proximal margin of resection, despite the Pathologist having reported otherwise at the time of surgery. What this meant was that all the cancer had, potentially, not been removed. This, by itself, poses a long-term risk for recurrence of the cancer, and, in the short term, would mean that Jack would need further therapy to try to ensure that the cancer had been eradicated. However, from the surgical perspective, a margin positive for cancer presents an increased risk for poor healing. Cancer does not heal like normal healthy tissue. The pathology report was explained to Jack and his family, and they were very understanding. It turned out that the Pathologist never actually performed the requested frozen section on the specimen. He merely did a gross evaluation; that is, he looked at the specimen with the naked eye, rather than under a microscope. His explanation was that he'd had years of experience and was able to accurately make a determination on margins based on gross exam alone. Obviously, he was in error on this case.

Things went from bad to worse for Jack. Three days later, he developed increasing shortness of breath and required endotracheal intubation and ventilator support. Shortly afterwards, he started to drain bile from the drainage tubes in his chest, which meant that some part of the surgery had not healed, and he now had a gastric pleural fistula, a hole in his stomach that was draining into the pleural space, which is where the lungs sit. He was evaluated with a CT scan of his chest and it was clear that not all the fluid was draining through the existing tubers, and a third tube was necessary. This was placed by our friendly Interventional Radiologist.

So there was Jack, on a ventilator, with multiple tubes coming from his chest and going into various body orifices. He had three chest tubes to drain the bile that was leaking, a nasogastric tube which passed through his nose into his stomach to try to keep the stomach decompressed, a jejunostomy tube which went through the left side of his abdominal wall into the small bowel to allow for feeding, a Foley catheter draining his urinary bladder, and a central venous catheter for IV access. A student who was present in the ICU commented that he didn't think any other tubes could be placed. This must have jinxed poor Jack because he next developed signs of worsening sepsis and developed tenderness in the right upper quadrant of his abdomen. Acalculous cholecystitis was diagnosed, and he had placement of *another* tube, this one a cholecystostomy, a tube placed into his gallbladder to drain it and relieve this source of sepsis.

Jack was quite a fighter, and he gradually improved. In fact, he was able to be weaned from the ventilator and tolerated the tube feedings well. The cholecystostomy tube was clamped, but the fistula from his intrathoracic stomach did not close. He improved enough so that after about six weeks, he was deemed strong enough to undergo another operation to repair the gastro-pleural fistula. Once again, this was done in conjunction with the Thoracic Surgeon.

This second surgery also seemed uneventful. The fistula was easily identified and was repaired in two layers and patched with some mediastinal fat. Normally, I would use the omentum, an apron of fat and blood vessels that is usually attached to the stomach, as a patch, but there was none available in this case.

Once again, Jack seemed to be on the mend until the seventh day after surgery when he started coughing. And, it wasn't just mucus he was coughing. Each cough left a yellow stain. He had developed a gastro-bronchial fistula, that is, his stomach had perforated again, only now it was draining into a bronchus instead the pleural space. His Pulmonary consultant performed bronchoscopy and was able to see that the bile was coming from the right lower lobe of the lung and that Jack had a very efficient cough mechanism that kept the airway clear. Jack, unfortunately, developed pneumonia and, once again, required ventilator support.

He received excellent pulmonary care from the nursing and respiratory therapy staff, and his overall condition seemed to be improved, even with the persistent fistula. Once again, plans were made for surgery. However, the day before he was to go back to surgery, he suddenly suffered a cardiac arrest and expired.

Jack also proved to be a learning experience. Whatever can go wrong often does. After caring for him, I changed my approach to surgery for esophageal cancer. I decided that it was best to stay out of the chest if possible, quite a trick, because the esophagus runs from the neck, through the chest, and into the abdomen. I started to do transhiatal esophageal resections. This approaches the esophagus through a neck incision and abdominal incision. The stomach is mobilized on its vascular pedicle as before, but the esophagus is removed by working up into the chest from the abdomen and down into the chest from the neck. The blood supply to the esophagus descends from the neck to supply the upper two thirds, while segmental arterial branches from the aorta supply the lower third. Thus, this approach affords access to all the blood vessels supplying the esophagus. And, because the entire thoracic and abdominal esophagus is removed, it is far less likely that the margin of resection will be involved with cancer. Finally, the esophagus is anastamosed to the stomach in the neck instead of the chest. Should a leak occur, it is far easier to manage through a neck incision than through the chest. Of course, the transhiatal approach is not always possible; if the tumor is growing into structures in the mediastinum and what is really blind dissection is not safe, then a thoracic approach would be necessary. For tumors that are not adherent to major structures in the chest, the transhiatal surgery works very well.

Sometimes, failing to operate or place a simple drainage tube leads to disaster. Bev was admitted to the hospital complaining of some nausea, something she'd suffered off and on for years. She had a large hiatal hernia, a condition that had also been present for years. She would be admitted to the hospital intermittently with similar complaints, would spend a few days NPO on IV fluids, and she would get better. She was high risk for surgery due to underlying cardiac disease.

This time she said it was a little different. She had a bit more nausea than usual and said she just didn't feel right. Her X-Rays were not significantly changed from previous films, however, and there were not any signs that suggested her stomach had twisted to the point of ischemia (diminished blood supply). However, because of her frequent episodes and her feeling that this was somehow different, I gave her the option of proceeding with surgical repair. She agreed, and the procedure was scheduled for the following day.

The following morning, I received a call from Dr. S, one of the Pulmonary specialists, informing me that Bev had been transferred to the ICU, intubated and was on a ventilator. She was not doing very well; as a matter of fact, she was in a preterminal condition and probably would not survive the day. It seems that she had vomited during the night and now had severe aspiration pneumonia. Needless to say, the surgery was cancelled, and she expired later that day.

Her case gnawed at me for weeks afterwards. When I first saw her, I considered taking her immediately to surgery. However, she didn't appear that ill, and there were no signs of ischemic or gangrenous stomach, conditions that would have mandated emergency surgery. She said that her nausea had improved and that she felt hungry; therefore, I decided that placement of a nasogastric tube, that is a tube passed through her nose into her stomach to allow decompression, would not be necessary. If I had done either intervention, it is likely she would not have vomited, aspirated, and died. Errors in judgment never sit very well, particularly when such errors cost a life.

A similar case is Walter. He was 76 years old and had lung cancer. I was asked to see him to place a venous access port, which is an IV access device that is totally implanted under the skin. Having only limited contact with the outside world greatly decreases the risk that the port will become infected. Walter went to surgery for this usually straightforward, uncomplicated procedure. The technique to place these ports is to use a needle to aspirate the subclavian vein, which is a large vein that runs underneath the collarbone. A flexible guide wire is passed through the needle and positioned in the superior vena cava using fluoroscopy to determine that the wire is properly positioned. Then the catheter portion of the port is threaded over the guide wire, its position confirmed with fluoroscopy again. Finally, the port is connected to the catheter, a pocket under the skin is created, and the port is placed into the pocket, held in place with sutures while the catheter portion traverses the subcutaneous tissues, and passes into the vein, with the end positioned just above the junction of the vena cava and the heart.

The placement of Walter's port was only a little less straightforward. I recall that the guide wire initially took a bit of a circuitous route to reach the superior vena cava and required some repositioning, but in the end it seemed to be positioned properly. I was able to aspirate blood from the device, usually a good indication that it is in a vein and the blood is not under arterial pressure, which would have suggested that it was in an artery instead of a vein. The next morning Walter started his chemotherapy treatment and all seemed well. However, the following day he was transferred to the ICU with fever and shortness of breath. I was called to come and check the port. I found Walter to be very short of breath, and I called for assistance, because I thought he needed to be on a ventilator. After this was accomplished, I checked his venous port. I found that fluids seemed to infuse properly, and I was able to draw back some blood, but the aspirated blood was not as free flowing as I would have expected. Still, I thought the port and catheter were OK to be used. Sometimes, the aspiration of blood might not be as expected; the catheter might be sitting against the wall of the vein or might develop a small clot.

Well, I was wrong. Walter became sicker with signs of severe infection. A CT scan of his chest revealed severe infection in his mediastinum, the part of the chest where the heart, trachea, esophagus, and several major blood vessels reside. It was decided that there was a problem with venous port and it was removed. Walter did not improve and he eventually died of severe sepsis due to mediastinitis.

I went through this case over and over again in the weeks after Walter's demise. I was pretty sure that the initial placement was not exactly where it should have been. I suspect that the end of the catheter migrated into a branch off one of the major veins. As the irritating chemotherapy agents were infused the small vein that the tip of the catheter was sitting in probably thrombosed and the chemo medication infused into the mediastinal tissue, rather than into the vascular system. This would lead to tissue necrosis and secondary infection.

I made several mistakes during this so-called simple procedure. When I saw that the catheter was taking an unusual path to its final position, I should have done something to insure proper placement, such as inject some contrast material to insure that the device was within a vein and within the proper vein. When I re-evaluated the port, after Walter became ill, I should have directed the ICU staff to refrain from using it and established new IV access immediately. I can make excuses as to why I didn't do this. I clearly recall that I was very tired the night Walter became sick, and I didn't want to take the time to put in a new IV line. This decision probably sealed Walter's fate. Or, I could rationalize and say that he was a sick old man with cancer, and this was probably why he died.

Finally, even the simplest surgery can turn into disaster. Robert was an 86-year-old man who came to the office with a cyst on his back. The lump had been present for years, but Robert said that it bothered him. It wasn't too big, and Robert was an otherwise healthy octogenarian. The cyst was excised in the office under local anesthesia and he was sent home with a few pain pills and instructions to return the following week to check the wound and have his sutures removed. Unfortunately, I had to see Robert much sooner.

I received a call from the ER that night. Robert was there with a blood pressure of 70/0 and heart rate of 130. The wound on his back was swollen and black, and the ER physician thought he felt some crepitance (air) in the tissue around the wound. I hurried in to see him and found him to be very ill. He had received two liters of IV fluid, and his blood pressure remained around 70 systolic. He was alert, however, and complained of severe pain where I had excised the cyst from his back. As reported by the ER doctor, there was crepitance in the tissue around the site of recent surgery and there was a black area about 8 cm in diameter and redness of the skin for a distance of about another 10 cm in all directions.

It was apparent Robert had a necrotizing soft tissue infection. He was resuscitated with IV fluids and given IV antibiotics and expeditiously taken to the OR, where extensive debridement of the dead skin, subcutaneous tissue, fascia, and muscle was performed. At the end of the surgery, he had a large open wound on his back, about 30 by 30 cm. He seemed a bit more stable with a blood pressure of 90 systolic, but required supportive care with pressors, and his blood was not clotting well. The large open wound continuously oozed bright red blood. Attempts to cauterize the bleeding were unsuccessful, and attempts to pack the wound were only marginally successful. Over the ensuing 24 hours, he developed progressively worsening multisystem organ failure and continued to bleed, from everywhere. Despite all efforts, he expired. He had developed a severe *Streptococcal* infection, the so-called flesh eating bacteria. Despite very extensive surgery, his body could not fight the overwhelming effects of the infection.

What did I learn? There's no such thing as a "simple" surgery. Even what seems to be a minor procedure can end in disaster.

.

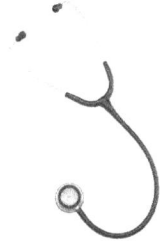

23. Monsters and Heroes

"There are no heroes...in life, the monsters win."
~ George R.R. Martin

In the practice of surgery, it is common for individual surgeons to try to establish a niche, an expertise that sets the surgeon apart from his colleagues. Some General Surgeons become expert in bariatric surgery, which is weight loss procedures, while others may specialize in surgery of the head and neck. In the spirit of increasing specialization, I've decided to concentrate my surgical practice in the area of tending to the powerful and famous.

I must clarify this, however, by stating that I don't refer to such trite and mundane figures as Presidents, royalty, sports stars, or movie icons. These media-driven figures offer no special challenge to a surgeon's quest for greater challenges, the constant search for endeavors that tax ingenuity and skill. The individuals to whom I plan to offer my services are the truly powerful: superheroes such as Spiderman and Superman; along with the elite of horror: Vampires, werewolves, and Frankenstein's Monster. Such powerful individuals present special challenges, challenges for which my unique skills and innovative talents are particularly well-suited.

For instance, let's start with Superman. Here is an individual, a refugee from the now annihilated planet Krypton. On Earth, he displays near invincible superpowers, extraordinary strength, invulnerability to all weapons, defiance of gravity, and many other traits. But, is he immune from disease? Does his reported highly dense molecular structure eliminate the possibility of gallstones or an enlarged prostate? I doubt it.

But, surgery on such an entity poses problems never encountered in the typical residency program. After all, how can even the finest surgeon begin to operate on a being that is impervious to knives, bullets, nuclear weapons, fire, and everything else? This issue actually was addressed in one of the Superman stories. The obvious solution was to have Kryptonite in the OR to diminish the invulnerability of the Man of Steel. From my perspective, however, this method lacks the necessary refinement inherent to most operations. It would be far better to incorporate Kryptonite into the surgical instruments that would be utilized during any operation. The smaller amounts of Kryptonite would make for an operation that is more controlled and safer for the patient.

What about other superheroes? The Fantastic Four, composed of Reed Richards with his ability to stretch to amazing lengths; his wife, Sue Storm, who can become invisible and generate force fields; Johnny Storm, capable of becoming a human torch on command; and Ben, a/k/a "The Thing," super strong and composed of solid rock; each would require special precautions and instrumentation should they need surgery. And, with the way they are out and about, fighting evil Dr. Doom and such, they are high risk to suffer serious trauma. I'll bet they can't even get health insurance, even under the impending Obamacare. But, I digress.

Surgery on Reed Richards probably would require a very sharp scalpel to compensate for his extreme elasticity; a laser could be more appropriate to cut through the elastic tissue. However, once the injured or diseased organ was repaired or removed, reconstruction would be greatly simplified. The problem of excessive tension on a repair or anastamosis becomes moot in such a being.

Sue Storm's special powers would require that she be maintained deeply under anesthesia throughout the procedure. Should she become "light," it's possible that any level of consciousness could trigger a reflex activation of her powers, and she could become invisible. I don't know about other surgeons, but I would find it particularly daunting to try to operate on an invisible patient. Of course, during residency, I did have the pleasure of operating with a surgeon who was nearly blind, but that is not germane to the current discussion.

Johnny Storm in the anesthetized state presents no particular difficulty. For my purposes, however, I would need to exercise caution if I were to use fluoroscopy during an operation on him. This is because I have a habit of yelling, "Flame On!" when I want to fluoroscope. It would be a pity if the OR crew was incinerated because of a lack of caution or slip of the tongue.

Finally, there's "The Thing," a lovable creature whose skin is solid rock. Once the incision was made utilizing a jackhammer, or, perhaps a diamond-tip saw, I suspect the operation could proceed unhindered. If, however, his internal organs were also silicon based, surgery in the usual manner might not be possible. A mason or stonesmith might be better equipped to deal with such a situation.

There are a host of superheroes who developed their prowess after being infected, exposed, or inoculated with some type of radioactivity, cosmic power, powerful serum, or other transforming material. Spiderman, The Incredible Hulk, The Silver Surfer, and Captain America fit into this category. They present the common problem of protecting the surgeon and OR crew from contamination originating from the patient during the surgery. Current gowns, masks, and gloves are no match for gamma rays and other types of radiation that might be percolating through the veins of these sometimes reluctant heroes. The obvious solution is lead-lined garb. However, such OR dress could greatly encumber the surgeon and lead to suboptimal results. These patients seem to be perfect candidates for utilizing robotic surgery. The robot's multiple arms would be safe from any noxious agents, and the operation could be carried out with minimal fuss. Once again, however, adequate anesthesia would be absolutely essential, as the robot bears a striking resemblance to some of the more dastardly super villains.

There are numerous other superheroes who present other potential surgical concerns, but I think I've covered some of the more important modern-day heroes. It's time to move on to the other end of the spectrum: Monsters.

Folklore, books, and film are filled with tales of werewolves, vampires, zombies, and such. Just as with the superheroes, monsters would require specific modifications of traditional surgical procedures, should an operation become necessary.

Vampires are all the rage these days. Vampire novels, movies, paraphernalia, and clubs are encountered on a daily basis. Are these forlorn creatures monsters, heroes, or both? I am not here to render judgment; I do believe that vampires would pose few serious impediments to surgery.

They live on blood, so nutrition is not an issue. Apparently, the blood can be consumed enterally or parenterally. They are universally described as pale creatures, suggesting they are chronically anemic and would well tolerate hemoglobin levels that are very low. Indeed, after being NPO for eight hours before surgery, it's likely that they would have very low circulating blood volume and low blood pressure, diminishing the likelihood of serious blood loss, even during the most complicated operation. Opinions on the effect of sunlight vary, but it would be prudent to operate in a room without windows to minimize the risk of the patient disintegrating into dust halfway through the procedure. Protection of the OR crew must also be considered. An accidental needle stick causing mingling of vampire blood with the surgeon's could lead to transformation of the surgeon into a state of being undead, like the vampires. I don't know about other surgeons, but my disability insurance doesn't cover such an occupational hazard.

Werewolves present an entirely different set of challenges. Tradition has been that werewolves can only be killed with a silver bullet, although more recent research suggests that it is necessary to completely dismember the subject to completely eliminate their existence. Thus, folklore suggests that silver instruments would be most effective for such creatures. Elective surgery should not be scheduled during a full moon, unless a qualified veterinarian is standing by.

Moving on, "The Blob" was a creature that came from outer space with a taste for the consumption of humans. Any attempt to undertake surgery on such an entity should entail caution. This beast would have no remorse at consuming the surgeon, nurse, or scrub tech. Surgery could only be performed using hypothermic technique. Such lower temperatures render "The Blob" compliant and eliminate the danger of being consumed. The anesthesiologist would be vital in such a situation, as he would be charged with keeping the patient's body temperature low enough to prevent untoward complications, but not so low as to kill the patient. IV access might be an issue, but I suspect a catheter placed anywhere into the patient would be adequate.

Zombies would not present any special challenge. They are dead already, their flesh is rotting and, in general, there are no operations that are actually indicated in this patient population.

Finally, no discussion of Monsters would be complete without Frankenstein's Monster. A being born of dead body parts, knitted together, and then instilled with life that originated with the powerful electrical charge of a lightning bolt. It has been stated, at least in film, that "The Monster" cannot be killed, that having been created from dead body parts, his life goes on indefinitely. Surgery becomes straightforward in this situation. Rubber gloves protect the surgeon and crew from any electrical surge, as they already protect us from the electrical charge of the cautery. Any injured parts can be replaced from the local morgue, although neurosurgery might require some delicacy to prevent radical alteration of "The Monster's" sweet personality.

There are other heroes and monsters who live among us, in literature, film, and politics (monsters only). Surgeon to such famous and powerful beings might not be financially lucrative (is any surgery financially lucrative these days?), but the experience, publicity, and subsequent fame should be fodder for books and TV appearances for many years. And, when it becomes time to retire, a tell-all book would sell millions, if not billions, of copies. "Does Dracula really sleep with a nightlight?"

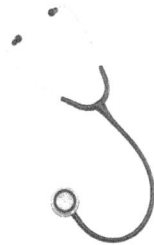

24. I Wish I Had…

"My motto is: Contented with little, yet wishing for more"

~ Charles Lamb

In the practice of surgery we surgeons utilize all sorts of tools to help us successfully complete the myriad of operations we are called upon to perform. Forceps, scalpels, clamps, retractors, sponges, electrocautery, sutures, and staples are just some of the instruments that are available to facilitate our task. There are, however, some devices I wish I had in my armamentarium.

Before every operation, the surgeon, assistant, and technician scrub their hands and don sterile gowns and gloves. The operating team does its absolute best to maintain a sterile environment throughout the case. It would be extremely helpful and would save a great deal of time if hospitals would install a "Surgery Pole." This pole would not be utilized for dancing; it would be akin to the "Bat Pole." Instead of the tedium of scrubbing hands for several minutes or using one of the newer scrubless cleansers, then waiting for the circulating nurse or anesthesiologist to find the time to tie your gown, the surgical team could slide down the "Surgery Pole" and emerge at the bottom scrubbed, gowned, gloved, and ready to go to work. It might only save a few minutes on each case, but over the course of a day, week, or month, those minutes would really add up.

The next device I wish someone would invent is a blood stream coagulator. During surgery, bleeding vessels are occasionally encountered, manifested by a stream or spray of blood escaping from the severed artery or vein. Time is wasted looking for the source of this bleeding, trying to follow the stream of blood back to the offending vessel. Imagine how useful and efficient it would be if all the surgeon had to do was touch the stream of blood and the cautery or laser or coagulating device immediately and automatically traced this river back to its source and sealed it. Surgical blood loss would fall dramatically, operations would be performed more quickly with fewer complications, and patients would recover more quickly. And, more importantly (at least to the payers), dollars would be saved.

The next item that would really make our operations simpler and safer is an anatomic identifier. There are numerous times during an operation when the surgeon becomes befuddled looking at a structure and wondering: "Is that an artery or a nerve? Is that really the Common Bile Duct or is it the Portal Vein?" With the Surgical Anatomic Identifier or SAI for short, all the guess work is eliminated. Not sure if the structure you're looking at is an accessory spleen or a malignant tumor? No worries, just give it a touch with the SAI and its powerful sensor will tell you in two seconds. Worried about biopsying that big blue structure in the neck? The SAI will put your mind at rest and tell you with 100% accuracy (or your money back).

During the preparation for surgery, after the patient is asleep, but before the skin is cleansed and the patient is draped, it is often necessary to shave the site of surgery. Actually, clippers are used, and this trimming of hair has nothing to do with risk of infection or obtaining a more sterile surgical field. The clipping of hair is strictly patient comfort and to ease the surgical procedure. Patient comfort because tape used to hold dressings in place tends to pull off hair when removed. Easing the surgery refers to keeping troublesome hair out of the way when trying to operate.

Because of the necessity that hair be removed, I wish I had a mini dust buster with a built-in shaver. Such a device would suck up loose hairs as they were clipped, keeping them off the patient and out of the operative field. Currently, the circulating nurse or assistant will take a roll of adhesive tape and try to gather all the loose hairs up onto the adhesive surface. This process is never 100% successful, and wayward hairs invariably make their way into the field, slowing the surgery and becoming a general nuisance. The "Razo-Vac" would eliminate this problem once and for all.

What about light? Operations are always done with some sort of illumination of the operative field.

Laparoscopic surgeries are done using a scope with a light that shines on the organs within the closed abdomen. Open surgeries receive light from overhead lights. These lights usually hang from the ceiling, are designed to focus their beam onto a fairly small area, and seem universally designed to frustrate even the most patient surgeon as he or she tries to properly adjust these lights to shine on the operative field of interest. Minutes, sometimes hours, seem to be wasted swinging these lamps one way or another, crashing them into each other (there are almost always at least two), finally getting everything just right, and then having someone bump into one or seeing it drift to one side or the other. There has to be an answer.

I would really like to see lights that move with me; lights that respond to my hands and head at, well, the speed of light. Move my head to the right to work on the hepatic flexure of the colon, the light moves with me; need to work on the spleen, the trusty light obliges. Surgery would be twice as efficient. There is a device called a headlight. This instrument of torture is worn like a hat. It has a light in front that sits between and just above the eyes and it has a screw in the back that tightens it down to prevent it from migrating, while providing the surgeon forced to wear this device with a good reason to go into Dermatology, as it bores into the brain. Once screwed into place the headlight, supposedly, can be adjusted to shine exactly where the surgeon looks. The problem, at least for me, is that it never seems to shine in exactly the right spot. So, I have to turn my head slightly. Now, I not only have a headache from the screw boring into my brain, but also muscle spasms in my neck from having to hold my head just so. Headlights and I don't get along. I'll hold out for the "Thought Directed Lightspeed Operative Field Illuminator."

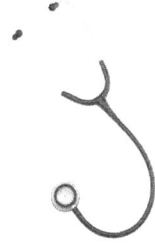

25. Ancillary Income

"Do not go where the path may lead, go instead where there is no path and leave a trail."

~ Ralph Waldo Emerson

Economic times are tough all around, and the practice of surgery is no exception. Falling reimbursement and a large population of uninsured patients make it difficult to make ends meet. In the true American spirit of entrepreneurship, I've decided to expand my business. Of course, saving lives and stamping out disease will remain the primary focus of my practice, but it's time for me and for our group, Coastal Surgical, to look for new revenue streams.

Let's start with something obvious, but, nevertheless, important and in great demand. Recent years have seen an explosion in the area of Bariatric Surgery, that is, weight loss surgery. The most popular, because it's a quick and safe operation, is the adjustable gastric band. This simple device is wrapped around the upper stomach and then inflated to constrict that part of the stomach and create a small pouch with a narrow opening. The patient feels full after consuming a very small amount and, over time, loses weight. This surgery is unique because the band is adjustable. A small fluid-filled reservoir just beneath the skin allows the band to be inflated or deflated, thus allowing more or less food to pass.

Currently, bands are adjusted in accordance with the patient's ability to eat or symptoms that might develop if the band is too tight. However, I think there is a huge market to attend to those individuals who desire the band be deflated for specific events. For instance, if portly Uncle Jack is going to his niece's wedding, shouldn't he be allowed to enjoy the large buffet, featuring all the lobster and prime rib he can eat? And, what about the open bar? What about poor Sadie, who has already lost 20 of her 400 lbs? Shouldn't she be rewarded with a night out at the Golden Corral? Thousands of our largest citizens are suffering under the torture of these devices. At $200 a pop, a huge market exists for the canny individual who seizes this opportunity.

A little shop on the corner equipped with an ultrasound machine and appropriate sterile equipment would suffice to provide gastronomic freedom to these sometimes desperate individuals. And, after the high school reunion or Bar Mitzvah, the band would require reinflation; another payday, perhaps at the discounted rate of $149.99.

Another new source of income could come from office souvenir shops. If you go to Disney World or Universal Studios or even your local art museum, the last part of the visit features a mandatory walk through the Gift Shop. Shouldn't a post-operative visit include a similar venue? After all, undergoing surgery can be quite a ride, and a souvenir of the journey certainly should be offered. Coffee cups featuring the Coastal Surgical logo, pens with blood red ink, or gallbladder-shaped wine glasses are only a few of the items that could be offered for sale. Plush stuffed organs such as liver, pancreas, or spleen would undoubtedly be hot sellers. Samples of actual organs, salvaged from real operations could be offered as collector's items, much in the way sea shells or various geologic wonders are sold now. Who wouldn't want the complete endocrine system, freeze dried and mounted for display on the living room or dining room wall?

Of course, postcards featuring images from actual surgeries would be available. And the usual coffee table tome, designed to impress the boss' wife would be on sale. *Colons and Hemorrhoids I Have Known: a Pictorial History of Coastal Surgical Group* is already in pre-production.

Beyond such souvenirs, extra income could be proffered from selling advertising space on the backs of scrub suits and/or white coats. Currently, I wear embroidered scrubs that feature my name and Coastal Surgical Group above the shirt pocket. There is plenty of space on the right side of the shirt and on the back to add announcements or logos.

"Miranda's Massage," if tastefully designed could be worn on Mondays, and "Joe's Diner" on Tuesday, and so on. I envision seven separate sponsors, one for each day of the week. There would have to be some discernment, however. "Evan's Slaughterhouse" would probably not be appropriate, unless the price was right.

Finally, the most lucrative untapped market is in the area of internal tattoos. Think about it; how many people do you know who have said, "I always wanted a tattoo, but I really wouldn't want to display it, or it's too painful, or I'm afraid of needles"? The obvious solution? Why, internal tattoos, of course, skillfully engraved on the stomach or liver or elsewhere. The bearer would have the quiet satisfaction of knowing he had a tattoo, just like his friends, without any embarrassment, should he meet that special someone years later and her name happened to be Lucy, not Sheila. Sheila would be safely tucked away inside on his stomach, instead of prominently displayed on his shoulder, and Lucy need not ever know.

A few cautions, however. For the man who tattoos a naked image of his sweetheart on his stomach; that svelte 36-24-36 figure would take on new dimensions after a very large meal when the stomach is stretched to massive proportions. General anesthesia would be necessary, but the latest minimally invasive techniques would be employed with minimal discomfort and no down time. I daresay that these internal tattoos would be less painful than their traditional cutaneous cousins.

But, the wearer wouldn't be able to see it, you object. No worry. Everyone who purchases an internal tattoo would receive a portfolio featuring his or her tattoo and surrounding organs in 4x6, 5x7, 20 wallet sized, and a 16x20 suitable for framing. Additional packages would be available.

Unprofessional you say, not dignified? These are difficult times for health care, with no relief in sight. These few suggestions are fully in keeping with the entrepreneurship inherent in the American Spirit. So, stop by Coastal Surgical Group, get your hemorrhoids checked, and pick up a souvenir mug on your way out.

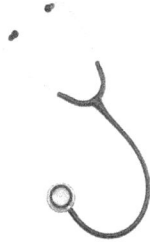

26. Looking Back

I've been in practice for more than twenty years. My patients have challenged me, humbled me, asked thousands of questions, complimented me, and criticized me, put smiles on my face, and made me aware of my own inadequacies. All the knowledge, skill, judgment, and perseverance that is brought to the operating room, along with a bit of luck, help bring the overwhelming majority of my patients to a successful outcome. Looking back, there are cases that stand out; cases I wish I could do over; do just one thing a little different, so that the end result would have been better. And, there those cases that amaze me, not because of anything I did, but because the patient healed perfectly in spite of all that happened.

Under the drapes a sick patient awaits, sleeping, filled with hope.

Glossary of Common Terms

Abscess: A localized infection characterized by an accumulation of infected   fluid

Acalculous: Without stones

Adhesion: Scar tissue that forms between organs, commonly developing after surgery or an inflammatory condition

Anastomosis: creating a connection between two organs or anatomic structures

Aneurysm: A weakened area on a blood vessel causing it to swell, which can lead to the blood vessel bursting.

Benign: a growth that is not cancerous

Biliary: Pertaining to bile, bile ducts or the gallbladder

Carcinoma: Cancer arising from epithelial cells

Cecum: The first portion of the large intestine

Cholangitis: Inflammation involving the biliary system

Choledochoscope: An endoscopic instrument utilized to visualize the inside of the bile ducts.

Claudication: Pain that develops in a limb during exertion which is caused by inadequate arterial blood supply.

Colectomy: Surgery to remove a portion of the colon (large intestine).

Congenital: A condition that has been present since birth.

Embolus: An object that travels through a blood vessel to become lodged in a distant organ, commonly a blood clot.

Endocrine: Glands that secrete their product directly into the blodstream

Endotracheal: Within the lumen of the trachea, usually referring to a tube in the trachea that assists with breathing.

Enteral: Within the gastrointestinal tract.

Exocrine: Glands that secrete their product through a duct into another organ.

Extrahepatic: Outside the liver, often refers to the bile ducts that are outside the liver, connecting that organ to the intestine.

Fistula: abnormal connection between one organ and another.

Gastroenteritis: Inflammation of the gastro-intestinal tract.

Gastroesophageal Reflux: A medical condition where stomach contents pass up into the esophagus, often causing heartburn.

Gastroschisis: A congental condition characterized by incomplete development of the abdominal wall.

Hematoma: Swelling due to a collection of blood.

Hernia: A defect in the abdominal wall that allows intrabdominal organs to pass out of the abdomen into an adjacent space.

Ileostomy: An opening in the abdominal wall which brings the ileum, which is the last segment of the abdominal wall to the skin level, most often necessary when the colon is diseased.

Incarcerated: Trapped, referring to a portion of an organ that becomes trapped in a hernia.

Intrathecal: Within the Central Nervous System, which is the brain or spinal cord.

Ischemia: A condition which develops when an organ has inadequate arterial blood supply. Excessive ischemia can lead to gangrene.

Jaundice: Elevated levels of bilirubin in the blood which can cause an individual to appear yellow.

Lacrimal: The gland that produces tears or the duct that allows tears to drain from the eye into the nasal cavity.

Lipoma: A fatty tumor

Malignant: A tumor that is cancerous

Mediastinum: The portion of the chest that is between the lungs.

Metabolic Acidosis: Excessive acid in the blood stream due to organs or cells producing too much acid or the body's inability to excrete acid.

Metastasis: A cancer cell or group of cells that has spread to a distant organ in the body.

Necrotic: Infected, dead tissue.

Omphalocele: Similar to Gastroschisis, a congenital condition characterized by incomplete development of the abdominal wall.

Ostomy: An opening created from an organ to outside the body.

Parenteral: Given directly into the bloodstream.

Pneumothorax: An abnormal collection of air outside the lung in the pleural space which causes the lung to collapse.

Psuedoaneurysm: A false aneurysm, usually swelling around a blood vessel caused by a hole in the vessel that the body has kept encapsulated.

Pulmonary Embolus: A clot that travels to the lungs.

Resect: Surgical removal of all or a portion of an organ.

Resuscitation: To revive an individual, usually by restoring or replacing essential elements, such as fluid, oxygen, or blood.

Sarcoma: A malignant tumor arising from connective tissue or muscle.

Seroma: Swelling caused by an accumulation of serum, which is blood devoid of red blood cells and most protein.

Strangulation: A condition where the blood supply to an organ has been compromised by compression, commonly found in incarcerated hernias.

Tamponade: Control of bleeding caused by compression, can also refer to compression of the heart caused by accumulation of blood or fluid within the pericardial sac, which surrounds the heart.

Thrombosis: The occurrence of a blood clot within an organ.

Tracheostomy: A surgical procedure where an opening is created in the trachea and a tube placed directly in the trachea to open an airway.

Vascular: Pertaining to blood vessels.

Ventilators: Machines that artificially breathe for an individual.

Volvulus: Twisting, usually refers to an organ that twists about itself, almost always a surgical emergency.

About the Author

Dr. David Gelber has been in private practice in General Surgery for more than 20 years in the Houston, Texas, area. He is a partner in Coastal Surgical Group and prior to this he was Chief of the Trauma Service and Director of the Surgical Intensive Care Unit at Nassau County Medical Center, Long Island, New York.

Dr. Gelber is Board Certified in General Surgery and Surgical Critical Care and is a Fellow of the American College of Surgeons. He was named one of "America's Top Docs" by Castle Connolly for 2008.

Dr. Gelber's other published works are *Future Hope, ITP Book One* and *Joshua and Aaron, ITP Book Two*, religious science fiction novels. More of his writing can be found on his blog, "Heard in the OR" at www. heardintheor.blogspot.com.

He has been married to Laura for twenty-five years and has three children, four dogs, and numerous birds.

www.ingramcontent.com/pod-product-compliance
Lightning Source LLC
Chambersburg PA
CBHW031956190326
41520CB00007B/268